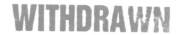
Praise for Dr. Rob's Guide

"*Dr. Robs's Guide* is good reading. He is one of the few broadcasters who have the knowledge of how important a parent-children relationship is and how it pertains to health issues...if you don't have your health, you don't have anything. Hopefully Dr.Rob and his book can help prevent someone avoid serious illness."

—Warner Wolf, ABC/ESPN Sportscaster

"Some are just born natural atheletes but others need some loving guidance at times. Dr Rob has crafted a masterful work—part survival guide, part instruction manual—for raising healthy and happy kids. Highly recommended."

—David J Shulkin MD, President and CEO,
Beth Israel Health System, New York, NY

"Dr. Rob's Guide" is a winner. This thoughtful volume is as timely as the headlines that warn about pediatric obesity, sedentary lifestyles, dietary deficiencies, substance abuse, and hurtful youth sports programs. These potent forces have combined to create a "perfect storm" threatening children of all ages. Dr. Gotlin's compact, readable, user-friendly book is stocked with advice for parents and coaches determined to stem the tide while assuring family-oriented fun and enrichment. The book's real winners will be boys and girls invigorated by sports and wholesome physical activity, led by devoted adults knowledgeable about health and safety at home and in their communities.

—Prof. Doug Abrams, University of Missouri School of Law,
Youth hockey coach since 1968

"Dr. Rob's book is a terrific way for kids and parents to stay healthy together."

—Billy Crystal

"Dr. Rob has hit a Home Run with this book. It is a "MUST HAVE" for every parent with a child playing sports."

—Mike Saunders, PT, ATC Former Head Athletic
Trainer, New York Knicks

"Every parent wants to raise a healthy child. Dr. Rob uses his expertise as a physician, coach, and parent to provide the blueprint of how to do so. As the mother of 2 young children, I will frequently refer to the many dog-eared pages of my copy of this wonderful book."

—Rebecca Lobo, Former WNBA Basketball player

Dr. Rob's Guide to Raising Fit Kids

A FAMILY-CENTERED APPROACH TO ACHIEVING OPTIMAL HEALTH

Robert S. Gotlin, D.O. (Dr. Rob)

Director, Orthopaedic and Sports Rehabilitation
Beth Israel Medical Center, New York, NY

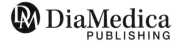

DiaMedica
PUBLISHING

Mount Laurel Library
100 Walt Whitman Avenue
Mount Laurel, NJ 08054-9539
856-234-7319
www.mtlaurel.lib.nj.us

DiaMedica Publishing,
150 East 61st Street, New York, NY 10065

Visit our website at www.diamedicapub.com

Library in Congress Cataloging in Publication data available from publisher on request

ISBN 13: 978-0-9793564-3-8
ISBN 10: 0-9793564-3-1

Note to Readers:

This book is not a substitute for the medical advice and assistance of individual physicians and other health care professionals who know you. Although the information in this book was developed to help you optimize your children's health and wellness, it is not intended to replace your own physician's medical advice.

Editor: Jessica Bryan
Designed and typeset by Gopa & Ted 2, Inc.

contents

Dedication

This book is dedicated to the millions of parents who want to raise their children to be fit and healthy. In particular, to my loving wife Marcia, thank you for supporting and standing by me in my relentless quest to better the lives of future generations. To my three loving children, Samantha, Adam, and Matthew, thank you for letting me be your coach, teacher, and—most importantly, your dad. Although my attention is often pulled in many directions, you understand my inner drive to satisfy the needs and demands of so many. You are my inner strength, and knowing that you are right there next to me keeps me going. I commend and thank you very much.

Acknowledgment

Being the youngest of three brothers, I learned early on that the family is a sacred entity. By assuring my safety and teaching me right from wrong, the lessons my family bestowed upon me set the stage for years to come. As a young child growing up in urban New York City, people in need always found a place in my heart. My father, my closest ally, always encouraged but never demanded my career choice of medicine. My mother, proud as could be, guided me toward good health and success, no matter what path I chose. The lessons of life my brothers continue to convey are always engraved in my thoughts.

For the past 17 years, Beth Israel Medical Center has been my second home. Without the support of Drs. Erwin Gonzalez and Norman Scott, the success I've been fortunate to attain might not have occurred. Valerie, my office manager, coordinates and organizes my complex life and schedule on a daily basis, and she deserves well-earned kudos. To Dr. Diana M. Schneider and DiaMedica Publishing, thank you for your professionalism, dedication, and relentless effort in bringing this work to fruition.

Assuring a healthy life weighs heavily on consuming a "good" diet. Without the insightful input and carefully designed "healthy meals" Toni Colarusso created, this book would not have been possible. Her expertise is clearly highlighted and the terrific meal choices presented will certainly gather the attention of even the "fussiest" of eaters.

About the Author

Robert S. Gotlin, D.O.

Dr. Robert S. Gotlin is the Director of Orthopaedic and Sports Rehabilitation in the Department of Orthopaedic Surgery at Beth Israel Medical Center in New York City. His practice includes orthopaedic, sports, and spine rehabilitation.

Dr. Gotlin frequently appears on radio and television, and in print. He hosts *The Dr. Rob Says...Sports Health and Fitness Show,* which airs every Saturday morning on 1050 ESPN Radio. He has served on the medical team for the New York Knickerbockers (NBA Basketball) and the New York Liberty (WNBA Basketball), and has consulted for the New York Yankees (MLB Baseball) and the New Jersey Nets (NBA Basketball). He is the Team Physician for the Harlem Wizards Basketball team, and a member of the medical team for Woman's Rugby, U.S. National Team.

introduction

One need not look further than across the kitchen table, to the other side of the classroom, or out onto the athletic field to see the results of one of modern society's biggest epidemics: the lack of physical fitness and its companion, obesity. We are "super-sizing" at alarming rates, and I don't mean just in the fast food restaurants. I am referring to right there under your shirt and inside your belt buckle. We are growing, not proportionally, but exponentially.

Certainly, media headlines have made us all aware of the alarming rise in childhood obesity. Statistics show that during the past 5 years, the number of people who are severely obese in the general population has quadrupled, and mild obesity has doubled. Nobody wants to be overweight. We diet, exercise, and follow gurus of every shade and stripe. But obesity rarely makes its first appearance in adulthood. It begins in childhood and is rooted in the physical and emotional life of parents and their children. *Overweight kids become overweight adults.*

Overweight kids feel self-conscious about their appearance. Frequently, they have behavior problems and are classic underachievers. Often, they are overlooked by coaches and teachers. We believe that the easiest and most effective time to address the problem is when it first begins—to prevent the childhood problems that being overweight causes and its effects that can last a lifetime.

In addition to the obvious obesity epidemic, children also suffer the consequences of misguided physical activity—sometimes too little, but often too much. Lack of exercise has its consequences, but too much activity also has its downfalls.

Parents, coaches, and kids need to be educated about the right mixture of physical activity.

This book addresses the questions most frequently asked by parents and coaches about children's general health and weight problems. We offer workable answers, especially as they relate to understanding the interaction between fitness and well-being, obesity and illness, and happy, healthy kids.

The challenge begins with recognizing the problem and then reclaiming our priority to strive for good health and fitness through regular exercise, good dietary choices, and structured family activities. We live in a hectic, success-driven world that often dampens our vision and sets the stage for future generations of illness and psychological turmoil. When 50 percent of elementary school children are reported to be either overweight or obese, when dads push their kids to play sports they have no interest in, when mom says "Little Johnny isn't too heavy; it's only baby fat, and he'll outgrow it," it's time to refocus our attention and address the epidemic head-on.

Being physically fit is not an option; it's a must. Consuming a good diet is not a suggestion; it's necessary for survival. I wrote *Dr. Rob's Guide to Raising Fit Kids* to alert families to the obesity crisis. This book offers practical, detailed solutions. Do you have a problem getting your son to eat a well-balanced diet? Does the idea of going on a "diet" cause emotional stress? We have the solution with our Power Sports diets. Your budding baseball star will dive into the Home Run Breakfast, and your young basketball sensation will welcome the Nothing but Net dinner. Our meal plans offer sensible solutions, with calorie counts included, to assist with proper growth and development.

We believe that fitness is a "family affair," and this theme flows throughout the book, which includes:

- Fitness guidelines for children ages 6–12
- Guidelines for selecting the right equipment for every sport
- Detailed meal plans that don't look like a "diet," as well as some great-tasting, healthy recipes
- Guidelines for children's exercise programs
- Advice for coaches and the parent–coach partnership

- A guide to common injuries and their management
- A discussion of how kids' health can be affected by drugs and alcohol
- A question-and-answer section that answers the most common questions

Because fitness is an ongoing effort, a companion website for the book, fitkids@ diamedicapub.com, has additional resources and an ongoing dialog to answer your questions, as well as a link to my own site, www.drrobsays.com.

Raising fit, healthy kids is not very difficult, but it has to be approached in a concise, well-thought-out, and consistent manner. This is the best opportunity we have to offer our young children a head start into a life of health and happiness. This book is intended to open our hearts and eyes to our children, who need us to understand them and their symptoms in a world that has grown increasingly manipulative and coarse. Healthy adults can help build a healthy world, and the routines for health begin in childhood. Together we can embrace a new approach to coaching our kids in sports, and in life.

Let's make it our goal to raise a generation of healthy young people who, through thoughtful participation in their world and sensible eating habits, will seek and develop their best level of performance.

⇨ *Success breeds confidence and confidence breeds success!*

chapter 1

fitness is a family affair:

RAISING FIT KIDS IN AN EXPANDING WORLD

Okay, Dr. Rob, we want our kids to be in shape for life, but what can parents do?

The first step is the most important: take time to consider your family's lifestyle. Are you always on the run? Rushing from a hockey game to a school play to a quick dinner? Hurrying to get something out of the fridge and into the microwave?

When most of us see an overweight child or adult we immediately think, "Wow. I'll bet junk food is responsible for their weight problem." In our rush to judgment we are only too willing to blame candy bars, potato chips, sodas, and plates of pasta for out-of-shape bodies.

Junk food, however, isn't the only reason we pile on pounds. *Junk lifestyle* plays a big role, too. We are truly a "sit-down society."

From the minute we leave the house in the morning, heading for school or work, until we arrive home in the evening, we sit—on the bus or train or in the car. Our kids sit at school all day long, and most of us have sedentary jobs. We come home exhausted, and all we can think about is relaxing in front of the television.

Studies have shown that there is a direct correlation between the hours of TV watched and a child's weight. It's important that we make our children understand we are not pushing them to exercise—but rather encouraging the healthy habits that will give them a lifetime of fun and energy. Exercising need not be a chore.

The most *avoidable* statistic is that more than 10 percent of children between the ages of 2 and 5 are overweight. Why this alarming increase?

It's not just about food. Think back to your own childhood. Your parents probably dictated the amount of television you could watch. Perhaps, as a parent, you also set time rules regarding homework and watching TV. But how does your child spend the rest of her free time?

When you were a child, chances are you went outside to play with your friends, because you lived in a neighborhood where no one worried about dangers such as child molestation. You *rode* your bicycle, *walked,* or *roller-skated* to meet your friends.

Many of us grew up in the "free-play" era, when you would pick up your baseball glove, grab the football, don your sneakers, and go to a nearby park. You either walked or rode your bike, yelling back to your mom, "See ya later." Without cell phones, this was the last communication you had with home until you came back for dinner. Mom went about her business and household chores, while you ran free and played with your friends.

It's different today, although it need not be. Fear has most of us closely linked to our children, and rightfully so. Concerns for safety are universal, in crowded cities and suburbs alike. We want to be sure our children are protected. For many of us, the best way to do this is to involve them in supervised play either at home or at the home of a friend. The backyard is generally as far as they are allowed to roam.

Playing with friends often means sitting at the computer text messaging or e-mailing the latest homework assignment laced with jokes. Today's youngsters average 5½ hours every day *sitting* in front of a TV, video game, or computer. This leaves little or no time for physical activity. Gone are the days when we ran to a friend's house to pick up something we needed or walked to the library. Author Rick Reilly says that kids today play "Sit on Your Can" not "Kick the Can." Most parents can remember pick-up ball games at a nearby field—today, those fields are covered with oversize houses—and consequently, we are looking at a lot of oversize kids.

If you think there's no cause for real worry because your kids are getting a full dose of physical activity at school, better check their schedules. According to an American Academy of Pediatrics Policy statement published in May, 2006, the availability of regular physical activity in school-aged children is at a critical (low) level. Although 80% of states do have physical education requirements for school children, almost half of them have exemptions from participation. The National Association of State Boards of Education recommends 150 minutes/week for elementary school students and 225 minutes/week for middle and high school students. A recent study of elementary school students revealed a total of 66 minutes/week of school-based physical activity, less than half the recommended amount.

Instead, school curricula are flooded with academic challenges, a focus on standardized testing, and blatant disregard for the essential foundation of academic success—physical fitness. Study after study supports the concept that physical fitness and scholastic success are directly linked. The better a child's level of physical fitness, the better his performance on standardized testing.

The result of this lack of exercise is evident not only in academic performance. Many of us who work with young children see the physical results as well. William Whitener, the artistic director of the Kansas City Ballet, reports that his colleagues have noticed that children beginning dance instruction have less coordination, rhythmic skills, body awareness, muscle tone, and stamina than their counterparts did 10 years ago. According to Whitener, "We attribute this overall decrease in physicality to the lack of exercise among youngsters. Children today are behind before they begin."

Our sit-down lifestyle often leads to severe obesity, which has the potential to kill us and our children. "The American lifestyle is toxic," said Dr. Karen Rubin, a pediatric endocrinologist and professor of pediatrics at the University of the Connecticut School of Medicine, in an interview with *The New York Daily News*. The increase in severe obesity—defined as being at least 100 pounds overweight—has quadrupled since 1986. Instead of 1 in 200 diagnosed as "severely obese," we now have the diagnosis in 1 of every 50 children. The Centers for Disease Control has reported that one in three kids born since the start of the new century will develop diabetes and is a potential candidate for heart disease, sleep apnea, gallbladder disease, and depression. All of these health concerns are rooted in childhood obesity.

A recent body of evidence also suggests that kids who do not get enough sleep tend to be hungrier and prone to weight gain. Children who get less than 10 hours of sleep per night often have an increased appetite, because lack of sleep alters the "hunger controlling" hormones naturally found circulating in the body. Forgoing a good night's sleep has adverse effects on many aspects of health and well-being.

How do you know if your child is obese? The old-fashioned way was to look at so-called "ideal body weights," which can be calculated by taking into account height and weight. Today, however, we have a more sophisticated measure called the *Body Mass Index* or *BMI*.

What is BMI and how do we measure it? The Pediatric BMI is a correlation of how a child's weight compares to his height. The higher the BMI, the heavier a child is for his height. The Pediatric BMI percentile calculation is a tool used to assess how a specific child's BMI compares to other children of the same age and gender. For example, if a child's BMI is reported as the 50th percentile, this means he is heavier than 50% of other children of the same age and sex. If the child's BMI is reported to be the 75th percentile, he is heavier than 75% of other children of the same age and sex. Many BMI calculators are available on the Internet. Simply plug in your child's values (height, age, and weight), and you will get his BMI. The interpretation of these percentiles is as follows:

If your child's BMI is reported to be:
- < 5th percentile: The child is underweight.
- 5th–85th percentile: The child is of "normal" weight.
- 86th–95th percentile: The child is at risk for being overweight/obese.
- > 95th percentile: The child is overweight.

Studies suggest that 60–65% of adults are overweight or obese, and—even more alarming—a recent survey of New York City schools revealed that 43% of the children in kindergarten through fifth grade are overweight or obese.

⇨ *For the first time in modern history,*
the average life expectancy of children is declining!

Diabetes, hypertension, and cancer are now a concern for kids because of the surge in childhood obesity. It's time to get kids "fit for life," so let's get them up and moving toward a healthy lifestyle.

Fitness Is Not Only for Children

Look around you. Overweight children often have overweight parents, and although heredity plays a role in bone structure and body type, lifestyle also contributes to the plump as well as the fit next generation. Adults spend too much time on the couch telling kids how to have better bodies and, of course, no child likes being singled out for his faults.

You have to do more than stand over a child and nag. As bad as you might think your child looks, your child thinks he looks even worse. We all know that obesity increases a person's risk for a number of serious conditions: diabetes, heart disease, stroke, high blood pressure, and some types of cancer. But what about the emotional problems that increase with the extra pounds?

Body image is so much a part of our culture, and it develops at such an early age, that most doctors are concerned about the overemphasis on the perfect body and the ways it distorts children's perceptions of themselves.

It isn't just 10- to 12-year-old girls who are worried about having supermodel bodies. One hot day, I told the boys on a basketball team I coach that we needed to divide up into two groups for a practice game. They all had different color shirts on, so I decided to have half of the players wear their shirts and the other half play with their shirts off—like the old game of "shirts and skins." Much to my astonishment, my seemingly innocuous suggestion was received by some of the boys with great distress. A few of those chosen to be on the "skins" team were reluctant to remove their shirts, and I realized they were embarrassed because they were overweight.

Recent studies suggest that obese children believe their quality of life to be as low as that of cancer patients on chemotherapy. Obese children have difficulty with any exercise or sports activity, and they often suffer fatigue and sleep apnea, as well as feelings of inferiority.

> ### Check your family's BMI
>
> - See **http://www.keepkids healthy. com/growthcharts/index.html** for BMI charts for children aged 2–20 years old.

Tips for Change

Don't announce to the family that "we" are going on a diet. Slowly and quietly *make* the necessary dietary changes. Enforce the notion that it's essential to consume healthy food, rather than engage in endless discussions about dieting.

Don't rush out and sign up your kid for multiple sports programs, thus placing the total fitness burden on them. Stand back and look at yourself and your children as a family. What are you doing *together* these days? When was the last time you all hung out as a group? Kids aren't the only ones who need play dates. Families do, too.

⇨ *Beginning today, you can eliminate your "fat family" and begin to create your fit family!*

Most families have two working parents, often out of financial necessity and, with the possible exceptions of family vacations or holidays, our time together is limited. Begin by arranging specific times for the entire family to get together, with the goal of making fitness a family affair. Isolating an overweight child and making him feel like he has special needs will only reinforce guilt feelings about his body and doom any program to failure. Let's turn off the TV, leave the computer on "sleep," and try a few family projects to get everybody in step!

The Family Walk
Begin with a once-a-week walk on the weekend. The idea is to meet consistently as a family and walk together. In the beginning, it's a good idea to have a destination in mind—it doesn't matter if it's only a stop at the drugstore to buy a magazine. Reaching a destination means accomplishment and gives satisfaction.

Speed walking should be your next goal. Begin to pick up the pace, but just remember it isn't a contest. No one needs to "win."

The Paired-off Walk
If only one parent and child is available, that's okay. Try walking after dinner when weather and daylight permit. I know it's tough when you finally get your child all to yourself, but stay away from questions like, "Why didn't you turn in your English paper on time?" Don't turn the walk into an inquisition. This should be a time to enjoy one another, and if no one talks, that's okay, too.

Other Family Stuff to Do Together
- *Washing the family car.* Every kid is interested in this activity, because they're all waiting for the day they get a license and can express their independence by driving.

- *Walking the dog.* A boring job, but somebody has to do it—and it doesn't have to be done alone. Remember, 30 minutes of walking every day (yes, even walking the dog) burns 100 calories.
- *A little aerobic exercise.* Do you live near a park? Is there a school athletic field nearby? Fast-walk there with your child for a game of Frisbee, catch, or a light run around the park or track perimeter—end with a few push-ups or jumping jacks. Even though it's a workout for the kids' benefit, you'll be amazed at how much better *you* will sleep.
- *A trip to the mall.* No exercise there? Wrong. All you have to do is park at the end of the mall where you're *not* shopping, and start walking.
- *An elevator ride.* How can an elevator ride provide exercise? It can if you leave the elevator for others and take the stairs. If you're going to the twelfth floor, press 10, and walk up the last two flights. Pick a floor between one and ten, and keep changing it for variety and cardiovascular strengthening.
- *Gardening.* Try weeding, mowing the lawn, or planting something. Your garden isn't the only thing you'll improve.
- *Martial arts classes.* Classes are probably available in your neighborhood, and they are particularly good for bonding between child and parent.
- *Family exercise sessions.* Take at least 30–45 minutes each week to exercise together as a family doing sit-ups, push-ups, pull-ups, jumping jacks, and weight training. (Working out with weights is actually good for young children; for complete information on safe weight training, see Chapter 3).

Where's the fun? Probably right in your own backyard, along with all the other good stuff in life. Parents are good at scheduling learning activities, but in addition to computer, dancing, music, and language lessons, make sure there's time set aside for play—good old-fashioned running and jumping with other kids.

Free play is best for your child, and games like tag, hide-n-seek, or choose-up sides contests—games that require fairly continuous movement—are good choices. If you gather a group of friends in a park or playground and give them a ball or two, they will figure it out. Before too long, they will be playing a game you might never have heard of before and having loads of fun.

Adults need to lighten up on their approach to family health and think about having a good time. Send your children out to play dressed appropriately for the weather—not for the blizzard that might come 4 months from now. Remember, when they are running around, they get warm, so don't overdress them either. When they are all geared up and raring to go, just give them a peck on the cheek, pat their sweet little heads, and tell them to go out and have a good time. In other words, *relax*. Let kids be kids.

Conclusion

The problem of obesity can only be changed by spending more time together as a family and participating in fun activities, eating a healthy, well-balanced diet, and following a regular schedule of exercise and other sports. In Chapters 2–4, we'll discuss exercise and sports in detail, and then we'll move on to planning healthy meals and sports menus.

chapter 2

staying in shape: exercises for kids

Exercise, Dr. Rob? Great, but how do we pry them away from video games and text-messaging?

Some people think exercise is only for grown-ups. They think kids are flexible, limber, and that simply being young is enough to keep them in shape. This just isn't so. The right exercises at the right age benefit everyone, provided these exercises are *safe* and *fun*.

The exercises in this chapter can be used to supplement 30–60 minutes of play most days of the week. This will help form the basis for improving aerobic capability, general conditioning, and strengthening according to the guidelines of the President's Council on Fitness and Sports.

When developing an exercise program, remember that children are not adults in small bodies. Our goal is not to create the next weightlifting champion or winner of the Miss America Pageant.

⟹ *The objectives of an exercise program for kids are to maximize flexibility, increase strength, and increase endurance.*

Volume and Intensity

Two important considerations in designing a child's exercise program are volume and intensity:

Some Things to Remember
when Starting an Exercise Program

- A thorough medical evaluation is necessary before beginning any exercise program.

- Your goal is to provide a program that is challenging, yet doable.

- Don't progress too quickly. *As kids grow, so should the program. Let the program follow the growth pattern, not the other way around. Don't expect your child to grow beyond her natural strengths.*

- The exercises should not cause pain.

- If possible, have your child exercise with a buddy. *You're not doing this to create competition; you're doing it so the kids have fun and get healthy—and don't forget, mom or dad can be that buddy.*

- Keep a workout log. *This allows great feedback, which is one of the best motivators, especially positive feedback. By tracking progress, we build confidence and, yes, confidence breeds success.*

- Allow enough time to complete all components of the program. *It's best to exercise at least 4–5 days a week, setting aside at least 30–60 minutes for each session.*

- Aerobic exercises are best for improving endurance. *These are exercises that increase heart rate.*

- *Volume* is the number of exercises and number of sets to be performed. Children should exercise 4–5 parts of the body per exercise session. If weight training is included, three sets of exercises per body part are recommended for each session.
- *Intensity* refers to the level of difficulty of each exercise, based on the amount of resistance (weight utilized). Let's not overdo it, parents. In case you haven't noticed, your child probably has a very short attention span, and the last thing we want to do is turn him off to exercise the first time he tries it. Choose a weight or resistance level at which the child can achieve success. For weight training, he should be able to lift the weight 12–15 times, using the proper form.

Stretching and Warm-up

Before exercising, I recommend a routine of stretching. Many adults think kids don't need to stretch because they are inherently "flexible." This is *not* so! Although kids seem to be more flexible than adults, stretching is of utmost importance because they are still growing. In humans of all ages, the tissues that hold our bones together (the ligaments) are very dense and not very pliable or elastic; they are like a piece of rope. As a child grows, the bones elongate, and this increase in length sometimes puts extra tension on these supporting structures between the bones. If a child doesn't stretch, the ligaments are pulled tight, and moving the bones becomes more difficult. Stretching allows the ligaments to become a bit looser and increase in length slightly as the child grows.

Remind your child not to "bounce" when he stretches. He should hold the stretched position for about 30 seconds, and then gently release the stretch. Bouncing can damage the ligaments and cause the muscles to contract erratically. *Dynamic stretching* is another good activity. This involves gently moving the muscles through a range of motion, which will help loosen them. This also offers psychological preparedness before beginning an exercise routine.

Of equal importance is a warm-up, which helps by increasing blood flow to the muscles and organs. The simplest warm-up is running in place.

Recommended Stretches

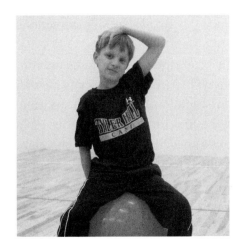

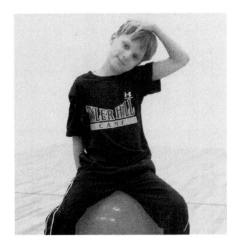

Neck Stretch. Sit on a firm, comfortable surface. Place your right hand under your right buttock. Then place your left hand across the top of your head and above your right ear. Gently push your head toward the right, while resisting the push of your head with the left hand. Hold this position for 4 seconds. Next, bend your head slightly further toward the left. Repeat by pushing your head toward the right against your firmly placed left hand above the right ear. Hold for 4 seconds. Next, repeat after tilting your head a bit further toward the left. After 3–4 cycles, perform the same stretches on the opposite side by placing your left hand under the left buttock, your right hand across the top of the head resting just above the left ear, and pushing the head toward the left.

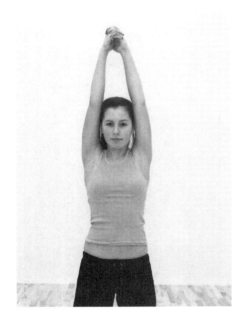

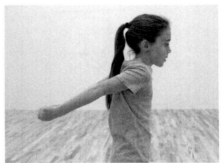

Reach Up (left). Stand with your feet apart at shoulder width. Extend your arms above your head and clasp your hands. Reach upward. Hold this position for 30 seconds, and then relax. Repeat 5–6 times.

Reach Back (above). Stand with your feet apart at shoulder width. Extend your arms behind your back and clasp your hands. Hold this position for 30 seconds, and then relax. Repeat 5–6 times.

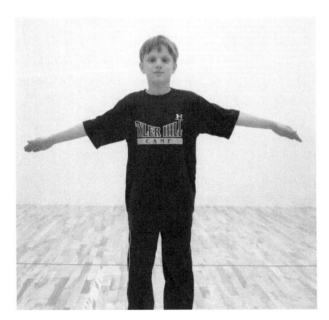

Arm Circles (left). Stand with your feet apart at shoulder width. Extend your arms to the sides of your body at shoulder height. Rotate your arms in small circles forward and backward for 30 seconds.

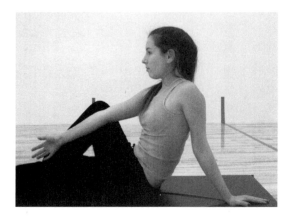

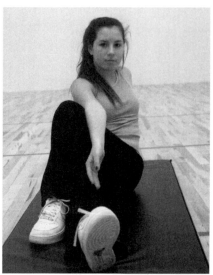

Low Back Stretch. Sit on the floor or another solid surface. Place your right leg out straight. Bend your left knee, and place your left foot over your right knee outside your right knee. Place your right arm across your bent left knee, and push your bent knee to the right. At the same time, twist your torso toward the left. Hold this position for 15 seconds. Repeat 2–3 times. Now, do the same stretch in the opposite direction with your right leg out straight and your left knee bent.

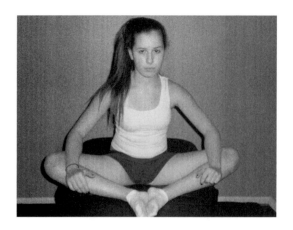

Groin Stretch. Sit on a solid surface with your legs apart, knees bent, and the soles of your feet touching. Gently place your elbows on your bent knees, and push down. Hold for 30 seconds. Repeat 2–3 times.

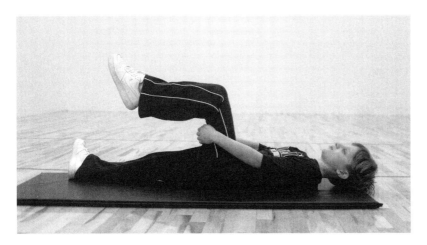

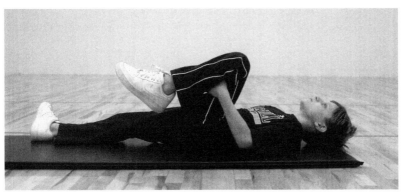

Knee to Chest. Lie on your back and bend your left knee toward your chest. Grab the back of your thigh just below your knee and hold this position. Try to lower your leg against resistance applied by your hands for 4 seconds. Bend your knee a bit more toward the chest and repeat 2–3 times Reverse legs and repeat.

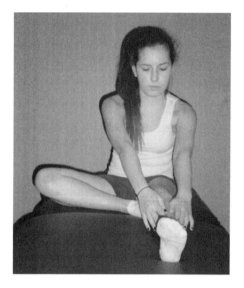

Hamstring Stretch. Sit on the floor with your left leg straight. Bend your right knee so that the sole of your right foot touches your left leg, keeping your right knee flat on the ground. Using your hands, reach toward your toes. Do *not* bend at your waist or low back; bend only through your hips. Hold for 20–30 seconds. Repeat 2–3 times. Reverse position with your right leg out straight and repeat.

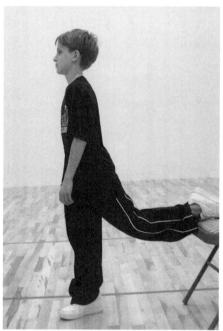

Quadriceps Stretch. Place a chair about 1 foot behind your body (the height of the chair should equal the height of the knee from the floor). Bend your left knee and place the top of your left foot on the chair. Thrust your hips forward while maintaining pressure with your left foot. Hold for 20–30 seconds. Repeat 2–3 times. Reverse the procedure with your right knee bent.

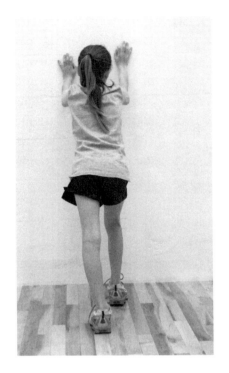

Calf Stretch. Face the wall, standing 8 inches away from it. Extend your left leg back, keeping the sole of your foot directly in contact with the ground. Gently bend your right knee until there is a stretching sensation in your left calf. Hold for 20–30 seconds. Repeat 2–3 times. Reverse position and repeat.

Recommended Exercises

Sit-ups. Lie on a cushioned surface with your feet flat on the ground and your knees bent to form a 90-degree angle. Place your arms across your chest, each hand on the opposite shoulder. Let the elbows rest on your chest. Sit up and touch your elbows to your bent knees, and then slowly lower your back toward the original position. Do this as many times as possible in 30 seconds. When this becomes relatively easy, increase the time to 1 minute. Keep this progression, going at your own pace, because this exercise builds strength and endurance.

Rapid walk/Run. Begin by walking at a rapid pace, and measure your progress by the distance covered or time of the walk. (A walk can be a predetermined length such as 1 mile or a predetermined time such as 30 minutes—either is acceptable. Kids of 6 and 7 years can begin by walking one-quarter mile; kids aged 8–9 can begin with a half mile. Children aged 10–11 can cover three-quarters of a mile, and those 12 and over can begin with a 1-mile walk or run.

Another good training exercise is the *obstacle course run.* Place several cones in a zigzag pattern and have the child run around the cones. This builds agility in addition to endurance.

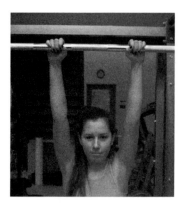 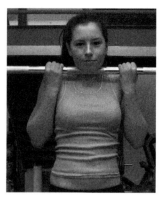

Pull-ups and chin-ups. Firmly grasp a bar secured to a doorway or parallel walls, and attempt to pull your body weight up, clearing your chin past the bar. Perform this as many times as possible.

Conclusion

Exercise is an important component of any program to improve the health of all family members.

⇨ *Get everyone up off the sofa or away from the computer and begin partici-pating in some form of exercise, right now!*

Useful Exercise Terms

■ *Aerobic capacity:* The ability of the heart and lungs to supply oxygen to the muscles. Muscles rely on oxygen as the primary fuel for physical activity. Exercises such as cycling, running, walking, and swimming help improve aerobic capacity.

■ *Muscle strength:* The amount of force a person can exert. The body has approximately 536 muscles, and each has a specific function.

■ *Endurance:* The ability of muscles to move for an extended period of time. Exercises that increase the heart rate and involve contracting muscles for a prolonged period of time improve endurance. Endurance exercises include jogging, push-ups, and swimming.

■ *Flexibility:* The ease of moving joints through a range of motions. The more flexible the child's body, the easier it will be for her to move.

chapter 3

sports for kids, ages 6–12

Okay, Dr. Rob, I understand that exercise and play are good for kids, but what about more organized sports?

Organized sports can be a real help in developing athletic ability and character. But, there's a confusing laundry list of sports choices, so here's some information to help you and your children make a decision about what sports might be right for them.

The decline in physical education programs in elementary, middle, and high schools means that parents must supervise at least some sports participation for their children. Individual or team sports? Which is best for your child?

Choosing the *right* sport for your child is of utmost importance. Children who are a bit more introverted tend to lean toward individual sports, and this is fine, but parents should also explore team sports. Both individual and team sports have characteristics that are important for the growth and development of children. It usually isn't the sport that scares away the child; it's the parent or coach who does them in. It's very important to evaluate and investigate the available leagues and organizations before enrolling your child. Be sure the level of competition is appropriate. Inquire as to the amount of practice versus playing in a game that the team or sport usually has (a ratio of at least 2:1 is acceptable). Attend a few of the games to see if they seem "right" for your child.

The goal of every parent must be to choose a sport in which his child can find comfort and confidence. It cannot be overstated: *Success breeds confidence and confidence breeds success.* For the younger child, choosing a sport or an activity at which he can achieve success is crucial. The sport and/or activity should not be one that *you* feel is important because *you* like it, but rather one that allows your child to achieve the intended goals: to improve physical fitness and learn the basics about coordination and skill. If you put a child in a program beyond his capabilities, everyone fails.

This is where a parent's judgment comes into play. Anyone who is responsible for a child's maturation must *honestly* assess that child's natural abilities. Learn what she likes to do and find the sport that best suits her needs and age. It makes no sense to sign her up for softball if she has no interest in the sport.

The primary goal is for each child to participate in a fitness activity that focuses on movement, coordination training, and the skills of sportsmanship. Remember, your child might enjoy more than one activity. That's okay, too. Some like weight training on their own and also playing in team sports. The *child's* choices will lead to success.

One caution: don't sign your children up for too many activities. I have seen parents who routinely enroll their children on several teams because *they* want the child to play on them all. This is not Mom or Dad's team, so cool it. Give your kids a voice. I understand that some kids need a little "push" or "jump start" to get going. That's fine—but don't push too hard. Allow your kid to be involved in the decision-making process.

Once your child is on a team, you can root for the team, check with the coach to make certain that the child's talents are being used and developed, and cooperate with other parents on rides to games, snacks, and other useful activities.

Please remember, *don't* overplay your roles. If you do, you'll get in the way of your child's success, dampen the coach's enthusiasm, and irritate other parents. During the games, the only words the children should hear from the bleachers are words of encouragement and praise for accomplishments. All kids need to be acknowledged in a positive way. Constructive criticism should come from the coaches during the game—and from parents after the game. It is always best to use this type of approach: "Son, that was a terrific play; great throw out there, but next time you might try it another way." During your child's developmental years, faults need to be corrected, but criticism must always be constructive, not destructive.

Just because your child is on a team doesn't mean that her exercise needs are being met. Playing baseball? You'd be surprised at the rather sedentary, low-intensity exercise your child usually gets during baseball practice. One of my concerns about team sports is that, although important things are learned, for many of the players, team sports all too often include excessive time standing around listening to the coach. Kids need to move. Coaches need to recognize this and be creative in keeping most, if not all, of the athletes involved all of the time.

Many social and family factors interact to keep kids from playing or participating in sports. Many of us have very busy schedules, the demands for academic achievement are intense, and the pressures of extracurricular activities fill the family calendar. It's easy to overlook a game plan that assures maximum health and fitness for the youngest family members.

Organized sports for kids are terrific because they teach skills that will bring pleasure throughout life and lessons in how to accept victory gracefully and learn from defeat. In addition, sports often provide the arena in which friendships can develop. Despite these pluses, team sports are not for everyone. Many kids avoid team sports in favor of individual sports such as tennis, golf, or swimming. Regardless of their choice, physical fitness is always the goal, not individual stardom.

The Fitness Triangle

No job is tougher than parenting. I know, because my wife and I are raising three children of our own. Fitness for children is about a triangle.

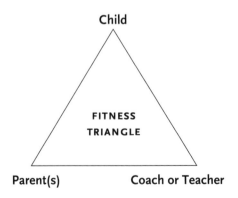

At the top of The Fitness Triangle is the child, of course. At the bottom are two supports: one base is the parent(s) and the other is the child's coach or teacher. These two supports provide the balance that keeps a child in top physical condition.

Physical fitness can be achieved in many ways, but children have the best chance of succeeding at any activity—whether as an individual or in team sports—when the three essential components of communication, cooperation, and compassion are present. Whether it's singles tennis or quarterbacking the Pop Warner football team, it is essential to maintain the fitness triangle. Team sports offer an opportunity to be a "member" of the squad. When a child is part of a team, some of his inhibitions can be allayed because teams win or lose as a unit. Fear of failure can be blended into the group; the spotlight never needs to shine on one child individually.

Team sports also teach discipline. I am a coach because I believe team sports teach kids basic coordination skills, emphasize the rules and how to play by them, promote thoughtfulness and concern for others, and provide the satisfaction of giving one's best for a common goal. Team sports offer the opportunity to teach sportsmanship, to learn from each other, and a chance for kids to feel comfortable interacting with their peers.

Team sports can also be a source of failure. Children who feel they cannot meet the expectations of unrealistic coaches or teammates sometimes seek refuge in an individual rather than a team sport. The concern is not so much which one they choose, but that they participate in some form of exercise or sports activity. Children and parent(s) should embark upon this task together, so make it a family decision. The child will want it and the parent (s) must assure it is "doable." That said; let's begin at the beginning on the road to fitness.

⇨ *I don't want to be one of those pushy parents, Dr. Rob,*
   but when can my kid take tennis lessons?
   Go out for Little League? Soccer? Lacrosse?

Slow down! If you think you might be pushing too hard, you probably are. Show me a 4-year-old who can hit a three-point shot, or a 6-year-old who can throw a curve ball, and I'll show you a parent who's dreaming about multimillion-dollar professional sports contracts and scholarships. I know you saw that 3-year-old hitting from the men's tees on the golf course in Florida, and who hasn't heard a proud parent boast of the preschooler who can pitch, bat, and spell all at the same time? Not unexpectedly, for most of us who have several children, this unrealistic enthusiasm and confidence fades with each successive child. It becomes rather evident that not all children can be the next Tiger Woods or Michael Jordan. The goal is to raise youngsters who will learn to reach expected physical skills within a reasonable timetable.

Growth and Development

Now, we are going to talk about *your* kid, your 6- to 12-year-old budding sports star, and what to expect in terms of physical prowess and emotional response. We are also going to talk about your role as a parent. Anyone who coaches knows that parents are partners in coaching, and sometimes kids think you are partners in playing, too. So, partner, here's the story on how your children develop at different ages. (You'll see that I haven't differentiated between boys and girls because at these tender ages their skills and aptitudes are similar.)

Age Six: The Restless, Fidgety Age

Because the attention span at this age is usually limited to less than a minute, games and sports should be about movement, not about "how to." Let your child repeat motions (throwing a ball, for example), and praise her for simply getting it in the right direction. If you start to go through the rudiments of baseball, don't fret because your son hits the ball and forgets to run to first base. The instinct for that next step (which is called *multitasking*) won't appear for at least another year. The concepts of time and numbers are just starting to emerge.

Your child might already know: "If I swing the bat easily, the ball will go a certain distance, but if I swing harder, the ball will go farther." While this is a key developmental milestone, it can become dangerous if the child is not able to differentiate "more is better" from "more might be less safe." This is the time to teach the potential dangers of power, including the random swinging of baseball bats in crowded areas. Unlike when your child was younger, you are now the counselor as well as the watchman.

Recommended Activities

A wide range of activities is recommended, because different experiences will help your child identify his likes and dislikes; try, for example:
- Kickball
- Skating
- Gymnastics
- Relay races to improve overall physical fitness

The Parent's Job at This Age

Help your child learn fundamental motor skills coupled with decision-making. Enroll your child in noncompetitive group sports or group movement classes. Offer praise even if the activity is not one of *your* favorites.

Age Seven: The Vulnerable Age

Suddenly, your child is aware that some kids win and some kids lose. He might not be thrilled by what he sees—unless he is the one winning. In that case, he will be very pleased with himself. If he is a consistent loser and the last kid chosen for the team, he will be heartbroken. Your job? Encourage, encourage, encourage. Even when it seems like throwing a ball that far is an insignificant accomplishment, offer praise. This is the time to teach your kids to reach for success. *Success breeds confidence and confidence breeds success.* Never expect kids to do things beyond their capabilities, because failure at this age is overwhelming. Multitasking now becomes a part of life. "Great hit. Now go for third, kid." The concept of "the team" also begins to take root at this age.

Recommended Activities

- Baseball/softball
- Inline skating
- Biking
- Kickball
- Basketball
- Lacrosse
- Ice-skating
- Gymnastics
- Fast hiking
- Swimming
- Soccer

The Parent's Job at This Age

Help your child experiment with various sports. Be certain the child has the proper equipment and safety gear.

Age Eight: The Age of Comparison

Now we're into that old question of: "Am I better than Jimmy?" The answer might not always please your child. Acceptance is of prime importance, and rejection often leads a child to isolate himself from group activities. Be ready with alternatives that your child can compete in with greater confidence. However, should a child's team be defeated, his recovery will be almost immediate. It's rare that a child retains remorsefulness after his team loses. It's usually the parents who dwell on the loss and replay the game at the breakfast table.

The Parent's Job at This Age

Watch for signs of withdrawal—this can be the first indication of peer rejection. Be supportive, and find alternate activities in which the child can be successful.

Age Nine: The Worldly Child

What other people think is more important than ever to 9-year-olds, but the over-involved parent now becomes both puzzling and embarrassing to kids. Competition begins to play a strong role, and at this early age we see our first sports dropouts. Individual sports participation begins to increase at this age, and children realize they have a choice.

They might be mediocre players on a team or possibly excel as a soloist. Remember, solo participation doesn't mean only golf, tennis, dance, or wrestling. It can be piano lessons, art, or language. This is a crucial time for parents. Pay close attention to your child's emotional reaction to all activities, guide him toward his best skills, and pay attention to his interests. Remember, Dad, kid sports isn't about you. Soccer moms might have to accept that their own dreams and desires for their 9-year-old might not come true.

⇨ *Parental pressures to succeed are very clear*
   to a 9-year-old, so don't push it!

Consider keeping a logbook on how fast your child can run or walk a specific distance, and offer praise for improvement. Children are ready for competition at this age, and the best way to understand competition is to compete first with one's self.

Recommended Activities
- Throwing balls through rubber tires
- Running races
- Weight training

The Parent's Job at This Age
Help your child concentrate on accuracy. Now is the time to hold a glove up and expect to have your child come close to this target when tossing the ball to you.

Ages Ten, Eleven, and Twelve: A Time of Fine Tuning
The concept of competition is now very real, and kids are ready to concentrate on individual skills. Motivation is high, and the will to win is present. Your child's attention span has increased dramatically, and he will listen to instruction carefully because this is the age when, if defeated, fingers will be pointed and blame laid, by others and the child himself.

By this time, children are well integrated into team or individual sports/activities. At this age, adult and peer pressure play a big part in the child's choices.

The Parent's Job for the 10- to 12-year-old
Look for programs and classes that focus on developmental levels (beginner, intermediate, or advanced) rather than chronological age.

Weight Training Can Begin at Age 8, Even Age 7!

Surprised you, didn't I? Weight training for kids? Not only is it okay, it's recommended. Weight training can be a terrific bonding tool in addition to improving physical fitness. I practice weight training with my two sons, and it affords an opportunity for the three of us to achieve a higher level of fitness, while at the same time being able to "boy talk" about "stuff." This is one way I can spend quality time with them, and I cherish the opportunity.

The misconception that weight training is bad for kids because it will stunt their growth is common worldwide, but there is little truth behind this myth. Weight training can be a good, if not great, choice for physical and psychological development in kids. As with any activity, the weight-training guidelines must be strictly adhered to. Although the positive results of weight training will become more evident each day, the prudent application of safety guidelines is a must. Although this is an individual activity, since it's imperative that kids don't lift weights alone, it is also a good way for parents and children to work together to improve strength, fitness, self-esteem, and overall well-being.

Even the American Academy of Pediatrics updated its policy a few years ago and reported that ". . . strength training programs might prevent injuries and enhance long-term health." The key in weight training, of course, is to use proper techniques and take safety precautions.

The most important guideline is the need for adult supervision. *This cannot be taken lightly.* An adult *must* be present and in attendance with the child to supervise the entire session. Kids can have Herculean illusions of grandeur. They often subscribe to the "more is better" philosophy and don't understand the potential for injury. Weight training must be well planned and precisely choreographed. Once the child demonstrates good technique and body posture, she is ready to embark upon this excellent activity for fitness development.

Let your child create his own weight training plan by keeping a log or diary of his activities, including the number of repetitions and weight level. Kids are often so eager to work with weights that they overuse them. Make moderation the keyword. The goal is to work 12–15 repetitions into a three-set series for each specific part of the body being worked, and *never* exceed 4–5 different body parts per session.

Your job? *Never* make weight training competitive. Be certain that the grips and weights are child-size. In addition to free weights, used no more than three times a week, you can devise an exercise program that mixes free weights with exercises that use the child's own body weight, such as push-ups or sit-ups.

Being on a Team Is Not a Guarantee of Fitness

Being on lots of teams does not assure fitness, and might even be an impediment to achieving it. I know firsthand that kids on sports teams usually get too little exercise, because they spend their time strategizing (no physical activity there) or sitting on the bench. Sure, a few stars play the entire game (not a lot of exercise, however, if we're talking about baseball and the kid is not the pitcher or catcher). My concern is that too many kids are sitting their way through team sports.

Beginning Weight Training

Weight training sessions should start at a frequency of 1–2 times per week. Each session typically runs approximately 30–45 minutes and incorporates 4–5 different muscle groups. The goal is to perform three sets of 12–15 repetitions for each part of the body being exercised.

The correct weight for your child is one that he can safely and effectively lift through a range of motion for all 12–15 repetitions, while maintaining good form. When in doubt, choose a lighter weight rather than a heavier one. When increasing weight resistance, add a maximum of 10 percent of the current weight or simply add 1 pound at a time. The weight is appropriate if lifting becomes difficult on the 10th or 11th repetition. If the child can perform all 15 repetitions with great ease, the weight might be too light. On the other hand, the weight is too heavy if by the 3rd or 4th repetition the child is using his entire body to complete the range of motion.

Weight training for adults normally stresses fewer repetitions and higher resistance. For kids, it's better to emphasize less resistance and more repetitions, using smooth, controlled motions. Like all workouts, your child should begin and end each weight-lifting session with 5–10 minutes of warm-up and cool-down exercises—anything from brisk walking to jumping rope.

Team sports teach kids basic coordination skills, the rules and how to play by them, thoughtfulness, concern for others, useful experiences in winning and losing, and the satisfaction of giving one's best for a common goal. Team sports are not for everyone, but at an early age, the social interaction and companionship kids experience is likely to be beneficial to most.

Keep in mind that younger children will suffer if undue emphasis is placed on the score or on winning. As a parent, it is your responsibility to understand the coach's technique and the effect that this technique will have on your child. Don't be afraid to speak up when you see something you don't like. Parents need to communicate with coaches so that, together, they can help a child succeed on his team. When approaching the coach, be genuine, courteous, and respectful. After all, he is likely volunteering his time and trying to teach each child the basics of the particular sport. The vast majority of coaches are earnest and fair. However, a few see only one player out there—their own child. It's bad enough when the coach's kid is the star player, and she seems to get unfair playing time, but it's worse when the coach "thinks" his child is a star player, when in reality she's mediocre, at best. Complaints in this instance are best directed at league officials and not toward the coach directly.

What About Girls and Team Sports?

With increased emphasis on sports for girls, many parents are paying more attention to the special needs of their daughters. As a coach, the father of a daughter, and a doctor, I am aware of the similarities and differences between girls' and boys' attitudes toward sports.

Many young girls share the eagerness and aggressiveness of their male counterparts. Others view sports as a social event. In my opinion, both attitudes are perfectly fine. Even before considering competitive team sports such as soccer and softball, your daughter might want to experiment with sports that emphasize her individuality, such as ice-skating and gymnastics. If she considers herself successful in this type of sport, she might never want to participate in team athletics. Or, she might want to move on from ice-skating and gymnastic competitions to competitive team sports. As she matures, your daughter will become more conscious of her changing body and the ways that sports and gymnastics can help mold it. All of us—parents, coaches, and kids—need to remember that the philosophy behind youth sports is the development of physical, psychological, and social skills—not to become the next Tiger Woods or Mia Hamm.

Conclusion

Be sensitive to your child's growth spurts, and help him understand that those suddenly big feet and awkwardness can be made more manageable with a fitness program.

Make sure that you and the other adults in your child's life are good role models. Do *you* have a fitness program so that your child understands that fitness is a lifetime commitment? A recent study showed that, in families where the parents were active, 95 percent of the children were active as well. Teach your child the physical skills that *you* should know.

Fitness begins at home, but it needs to be reinforced outside the home through supervised sports, and especially through school recreational and sports programs. Go to your school or board of education and petition authorities to add age-appropriate, fun physical activities.

⇨ *Mix it up. Have a good time. Exercise isn't just about getting fit; it's also about having fun!*

If your child is participating in at least 30–45 minutes of physical activity 4 or more days of the week, he is meeting the minimum suggested guidelines for physical fitness and is certainly on the right track.

chapter 4
the right equipment for every sport

Hey, Dr. Rob, there are so many choices at the athletic store. How do I know the right things to buy for my kids?

The first responsibility of a parent whose child is going to play team sports is to make sure your kid has the right equipment. By "right equipment" I mean both the basic equipment, such as bats, balls, and rackets, as well as protective gear when necessary.

When you and your child go to the sporting goods store, listen to her, but let the final decision be yours. No kid ever wants anything marked "Sale," and who wants to wear sneakers without a brand name logo? It's up to you to make sure that you get proper value for every dollar spent.

Unless your child is truly committed to a sport, it's always a good idea to start with the least expensive yet safe equipment. Remember, kids are fickle, and the enthusiasm for a sport might not last past the current season. If it does, there's always next year, when she will need larger sizes anyway.

Safety First

Let's begin the discussion of equipment with *safety*:

Sports in which the feet are not directly on the ground—such as rollerblading, skiing, snowboarding, or bicycling—are generally the riskiest and carry the greatest possibility for head injury. Therefore, *helmets* are essential. Although wearing a helmet does not guarantee the child will not have *any* injury should she fall, helmets do lessen the likelihood of serious injury.

When shopping for a helmet, don't be fooled by the color, the style, or a smooth-talking salesperson. Make sure the helmet fits snugly, with the straps forming a "v" around the ear. There should be no more than 2 inches of space between the eyebrows and the rim of the helmet. It's best to ask for assistance and have a skilled salesperson properly fit the helmet.

Also, for the sake of safe play, *buy proper shoes*. The best time to buy either athletic or everyday shoes is at the end of the day (or after a running event) when the child's feet are the largest. Shoes should always be fitted when the child is standing and wearing sports-specific socks. Make sure the heels fit snugly and that there is about half an inch of wiggle room from the end of the child's longest toe to the inside of the shoe. Shoes should be comfortable when your child tries them on, and she should not need to "break them in."

Basic Equipment

Now let's look at some individual sports equipment needs:

Baseball

Needed: Glove, bat, athletic supporter (for boys), cleats, batting helmet, and batting gloves

Buying Guide

The Bat. When you buy a bat, you will hear the word *differential*. This refers to the difference (in whole numbers) between the weight of the bat and its length. If a bat weighs 31 ounces and is 21 inches long, the differential is 10 (31 – 21 = 10). Bats for younger ballplayers have the largest differential (10–12) but, by the time your youngster is in high school, the differential will not exceed 5.

In buying a bat, consider its length, weight, and barrel size. Lighter-weight bats are best for kids 6–12. *Quick tip:* Using the outstretched arm of the dominant hand, have your child hold the bat to the side at shoulder height. If he can maintain this position steadily for a minimum of 20 seconds, the bat is okay. If, however, he gets "the arms shakes," the bat is probably too heavy. A good guide is:

- Ages 6–7: 15–16 ounce bat, 24–28 inches in length with a 2¼-inch barrel
- Ages 8–9: 15–17 ounce bat, 27–29 inches in length with a 2¼-inch barrel

- Age 10: 16–18 ounce bat, 28–30 inches in length with a 2¼-inch barrel
- Age 11: 17–18 ounce bat, 29–30 inches in length with a 2¼–2⅝-inch barrel
- Age 12: 18–20 ounce bat, 30–32 inches in length with a 2¼–2¾-inch barrel

The Glove. A child's first glove should be user-friendly—comfortable, soft, pliable, and not too big. Remember, all you shopping adults, using a bigger glove does *not* mean the little kid will make more catches. In fact, the opposite is true, because an oversize glove is too difficult to control, particularly for a young child.

Glove sizes range from 9–13, which is the length from the heel of the glove to the top of the longest finger or webbing. Infielders use smaller sizes (9–11); outfielders go for larger sizes (11–12); and younger athletes with small hands might find that size 9–11 is good for all positions.

The pocket of the glove should be deeper for an outfielder, and shallower for an infielder. For softball, deeper pockets are best.

Webbing is usually closed for outfielders (better support) and open for infielders (easier to get the ball out of the glove).

Here's what the sporting goods store *can't* do for your kids: break in the glove. That takes use, lots of use. Of course, the store will try to sell you oils, solutions, and creams to help, but nothing replaces using a new glove.

Basketball

Needed: A mouth guard is highly recommended because elbows and hands are constantly flying, and pushing and shoving are common.

Buying Guide

Footwear. Consider good ankle support to reduce the risk of sprains. Unless the child has had an injury, his ankles need not be taped, but be sure his basketball sneakers provide good ankle support.

The ball. Consider good ankle support to reduce the risk of sprains. Unless the child has had an injury, his ankles need not be taped, but be sure his basketball sneakers provide good ankle support.

Basketball Sizing

Age	Basketball Type	Basketball size	Basketball Circumference (inches)	Basketball Weight (ounces)
Boys & girls 7 and under	Mini	3	22-22.5	10.5-11.5
Boys & girls 8-11	Junior/ Intermediate	5	27.25-27.75	14-18
Girls 12 and older	Official Women	6	28.5	18-20
Boys 12 and older	Regulation	7	29.5	20-22

Soccer

Needed: Soccer shoes, cleats (or turf shoes), ball, and shin guards

Buying Guide

Footwear. Footwear is often referred to as *soccer shoes* or *soccer cleats*. There are two basic types, molded and detachable.

Molded shoes have nonremovable rubber or hard plastic formed to the bottom of the shoe for traction and control. This type is best for beginning and intermediate players.

For players between the ages of 9 and 12, it is important to look for an adequate number of cleats in the heel, regardless of the type of footwear you select. If there are too few cleats to support the heel, the player will have increased heel pressure, which can lead to pain and tendonitis. Also, to minimize the risk of ankle and knee injuries, younger players should not have any cleats longer than half an inch.

Turf shoes are a popular alternative to soccer cleats. They have raised patterns on the bottom instead of studs, and are considered very good footwear for hard, outdoor surfaces and on artificial turf. Depending on the raised pattern, some turf shoes can even be used in damp conditions. In general, they are a good all-around training shoe that can be used in games on particularly hard surfaces.

Soccer shoes are available in leather and synthetic materials. For beginners and intermediates, consider synthetic. Although you will sacrifice some flexibility and feel, its lower cost makes it attractive. Soccer shoes are designed to be a little narrower than everyday sneakers, but be certain that the shoes are not so tight that they choke the blood supply to the foot and are uncomfortable. Don't rush when buying these shoes, and have your child try more than one pair for comparison.

Shin Guards. If you play soccer, you *must* wear shin guards, which are designed to reduce injuries by absorbing the impact of players' kicks.

Many shin guards have attached protectors for the ankle and Achilles tendon. I strongly recommend this type for players under the age of 13.

Some shin guards are simply worn inside the sock, but these can slip while playing and some kind of strap is recommended. Some have Velcro™-type straps that wrap around the back of the leg for an adjustable closure. These are convenient and popular with players. For very young children, some parents prefer to sew the shin guard and ankle guard into a thin nylon sock.

Shin guards should weigh no more than 6 ounces (less than 5 ounces is preferred). They will probably cost about $15.

Soccer Balls. There are three factors to consider when purchasing a soccer ball: size, color, and quality.

Size 3 balls, which are 23–24 inches in circumference and weigh 11–12 ounces, are for young children under the age of 8.

Size 4 balls, 25–26 inches in circumference and weighing 12–13 ounces, are generally used for players age 8–12.

Size 5 soccer balls, 27–28 inches in circumference and weighing 14–16 ounces, are generally used for players age 13 and older.

The color and design will depend on your child's choice. Soccer balls tend to scatter during practices, so it might be a good idea to select a unique design or color so your child's ball can be retrieved easily.

Price and quality run the gamut from cheap plastic balls that are uncomfortable to kick to very expensive leather balls. Prices range from $10 to $50, with the main features being cover, panels, lining, and bladder.

Which one is best for your child or your child's team? It depends on both needs and resources. For most players, a polyurethane cover with machine-stitched panels and at least three layers of cotton and polyester lining with a butyl bladder should be adequate. As with all athletic equipment, the quality of the equipment can increase with the child's age, skill, and passion.

Tennis
Buying Guide

The Racquet. Beginners should look for a basic racquet. In general, oversized pre-strung racquets provide the greatest versatility and have the largest sweet spots, a real plus for beginners.

Intermediate players need a racquet that will complement their game. If the player is a hard hitter, a lighter and smaller racquet is best because it gives greater control.

Advanced players want high-tech, composite racquets that are more expensive but offer superior power and control.

The standard guide for children is:

- 4 years of age: 19-inch racquet
- 4–6 years: 21-inch racquet
- 7–8 years: 23-inch racquet
- 9–10 years: 25-inch racquet
- 10–12 years: 26-inch racquet

Remember, this is a guide, not a mandate. You can adjust the size based on your child's size and experience.

The racquet shape involves two factors: look and feel. An oval racquet is traditionally thought to offer a superior feel, with its sweet spot in the bottom half. The teardrop racquet has a larger sweet spot, and is considered more practical for beginners.

The grip size is crucial. The ideal size is the distance from the middle of the palm to the tip of the ring finger.

For beginner and many intermediate players, pre-strung racquets are the most affordable, versatile, and practical. The thickness of the string is another consideration. Thicker strings (15-gauge) last longer but do not feel as good as thinner strings (16- and 17-gauge).

Conclusion

Sports equipment that is designed well for safety and sized correctly will assure your child of success, and success brings confidence.

chapter 5

advice for coaches: the parent partnership

Dr. Rob, I'm a parent and coach—just like you. Please give us coaches some advice, and how about a few words for those cheering on the sidelines?

There are more than two million volunteer youth coaches in the United States, and my guess is that most of them have not had any formal training in coaching. Most parent-coaches are out there because our kids want to play (or we think they should), and we regard coaching as a great way to bond with our children.

Parental involvement has steadily increased. We welcome it, and we also recognize that with it come responsibilities and a need for understanding just what is expected of a volunteer coach. The definition of a good coach is to be a good *teacher*. This is best explained through a few stories:

We were assigning players to teams in our kids' basketball league, when Jack, one of the coaches, said, "I'll take Billy. His dad told me he wants him on my team. Besides, I can carpool him to the games."

Most of us smiled. We knew Jack was pushing hard for Billy—not for the reasons he had given, but because Billy was touted to be the best player in the league that year.

The next name requested was Terry. "I'll take him," said Brad, another coach.

"Terry?" Jack laughed. "That kid doesn't know one end of the basketball court from the other. Why do you want him?"

Brad put down his pencil and looked at Jack. "I had Terry last season," he said.

"And although we didn't win the championship, or even come in second, Terry played his heart out. After the last game, his dad wrote and thanked me because Terry had repeatedly told him he'd rather play with our team and lose than win a championship. He liked his teammates and the way he was treated. This was the first team he had played on where he felt accepted and like he belonged, and where his contribution was valued."

Nobody said anything much after that, but later I told Brad how strongly I agreed with him. This is what coaching is all about.

Eight Tips for Successful Coaching

1. Listen to your players. Kids don't always use words to express themselves, and a good coach knows his players well enough to hear them even when they don't say anything. Body language tells a lot.
2. Remember each kid's name early on. It builds confidence and trust between player and coach.
3. Acknowledge effort as much as results. An encouraging word early in the season helps a player feel like part of the team.
4. Hold a team meeting early in the season, and tell the parents about your coaching style and your expectations of them—as well as their kids.
5. Plan each practice session and make it fun and creative; be sure to involve all the kids most of the time.
6. Mix up the drills, and give the kids a "fun break" somewhere during the practice. This could be a kicking contest, relay race, or free-throw shooting competition.
7. Focus on the child's skills when the two of you are interacting. Always emphasize what the child does well, and don't expect a performance that exceeds her skill levels.
8. Clearly state your practice goals and expectations, because the players must understand that these games are not for parents and coaches. Tell them, "Hey, kids, this is all about YOU."

A lot of adults who coach kids forget that coaching is about the life lessons we can teach children through sports. A good coach needs to be a good teacher because, until the age of 12, coaching is all about teaching—teaching the rules, teaching acceptance of the strengths and weaknesses of self and others, and teaching kids how to play by the rules. Unfortunately, there's a whole lot of coaches who expect to live the game day after day, night after night, week after week. These are the coaches who want to strategize every play, and replay every game for weeks after they're over.

⇨ *Young kids are not looking to play war games!*

It's the win-at-all-costs mentality of so many coaches (who take their cues from the professional coaching ranks) that takes most of the fun out of youth sports. When we step onto the playing field, some of us tend to forget that the youngsters we're coaching are simply kids who like to play, and it doesn't much matter if it's Game Boy or youth sports. Kids just want to have fun. When the game is over, they pick themselves up and go on to the next thing that interests them. It's the coach who can't get over the losses, and who can't accept the wins without assuming that she made them happen.

I can't say this often enough: adults who coach kids under the age of 13 must teach them to trust themselves and have confidence in their own abilities, and to know the rewards of feeling they've done their best.

What Makes a Successful Coach?

All successful coaches have one quality in common: they are able to identify at least one talent in each team member, and then help the child work on, improve, and reap the rewards of their talent.

If the game is basketball, it might mean taking the gawky, tall kid with a knack for blocking shots (or at least distract a shooter) and help him feel less awkward on the court and less clumsy in life.

In baseball, the successful coach is able to work with the little guy who might not be the greatest hitter but can reach first base on a walk.

A good coach shines a tiny spotlight on every contribution made by the classic underachievers and recognizes them along with all the other kids after the game. That's how good coaches teach team spirit and sportsmanship.

The Parent Partnership

Most adults who coach kids' teams are parents, and sometimes we look at the other parents who come to our games and we can't believe our eyes. We all know the moms who come to the games and spend their time on their cell phone talking to their friends or gossiping with the other moms in the stands. We recognize the dads who do the same thing, chatting about the recent major league baseball game rather than watching their kid play. When the game ends, they are never sure who won.

On the other hand, I often see the frustrated coach who is unable to get an eager dad off the sidelines of a baseball game. The parent who thinks he has to tell his son where to stand in the outfield, how to bat, and when to run; throughout the game, this dad constantly shouts instructions to his kid, which are often in conflict with the directions given by the coach.

Given a choice, I think I'd take the cell-phoners ("the cellers") over the passionate parents ("the yellers"). When the "bleacher mom or dad" is competing with the coaching staff for a player's attention, the result for the athlete is almost always confusion. It's difficult enough for a young child to process directions from the coaching staff, but when a second set of directives is coming from mom and/or dad, failure is assured.

Then we have the parents who doubt everything the referee or umpire says. Some parents don't even realize how obnoxious they are, once they start second-guessing the game officials. One day, at a soccer game in suburban Cleveland, teenaged Stephanie was refereeing the pigtail game when two girls from opposing teams collided on the field. Both fell to the ground and, when one got up and one stayed on the ground crying, Stephanie blew her whistle, stopped the game, and rushed to help the crying girl.

The girl's father ran onto the field, and Stephanie breathed a sigh of relief because, obviously, he was there to care for her. But instead of assisting his daughter, the father waved his arms and screamed at Stephanie. "Are you blind? You girls are stupid," he shouted at the young referee. The head of the recreational sports depart-

How to Be a Supportive Parent

- Go to the games—and sometimes the practices.
- When you're at the game, cheer for both teams and show enthusiasm for any kids who perform well, including your own.
- Be respectful of the physical surroundings. Don't litter.
- Be respectful of all the players. Don't make disparaging remarks about any players—yours or theirs.
- Don't coach from the sidelines. One coach is enough for any team.
- Stay off the field unless there is an injury you can help with, and always announce who you are when offering help.
- Don't pressure your kid to succeed, because success is not what you might think it is. A kid who comes off the field thinking he had a great time with pals and maybe even helped with the win—or kept the loss from being greater—is the true success.
- Don't embarrass your child by offering advice when it isn't necessary—particularly to the coach or other parents.
- Talk to your child after the game and check his enjoyment level, self-esteem, respect for his peers and coaches, and teamwork. Talk to the coach if you hear about or notice a problem. (No one ever beat Mom or Dad in recognizing the first signs of trouble.)
- Your kid might never score a goal, hit a home run, or hold back the other team. *But,* if he is as pleased with himself as the kids who did, you're doing something right

ment happened to be present, and he stopped the game and escorted the father from the field. He told the father he would not be permitted to attend any future games. The father was so angry that he withdrew his daughter from the league.

The player and her father were not the only emotional victims that afternoon.

Visibly shaken, Stephanie told her parents that she didn't want to referee anymore if she had to deal with that kind of abusive behavior from adults. They assured her that the pigtailer's father would soon come to his senses and apologize, but he didn't.

Several weeks later, Stephanie's parents met the belligerent dad at a party and informed him that it was *their* daughter he had berated at the soccer game. Now embarrassed by his irrational behavior, the father called the teenager and offered his apology. For Stephanie, it was "too little, too late." She had already stopped refereeing.

Coaches sometimes have a tough time when their own kids are on the team. That's why I like this story about resolving conflicting emotions. It comes from Matt Levine of New York, who coaches a Doc's NYC Youth Lacrosse team. Matt's fifth grade son was one of the starting players on the defense. At one point during the game, the boy stormed off the field and had harsh words with his father. This caused the boy to respond with a typical kid reaction—he didn't want to play anymore.

Matt looked at the watchwords of the league, which appear on the backs of all the kids' lacrosse t-shirts: "Honor the Game." Matt turned to his son and said, "Okay. The best thing we can do right now is to Honor the Game, both of us. This game is bigger than the coach arguing with one of his players."

This cooled down the emotions of both father and son, and eventually the boy said he was ready to go back into the game.

"We both finished up the day's tournament on a good note," Matt said. "And this added to my effectiveness in coaching the rest of the team. I have invoked Honor the Game at other tense moments with my son. It works best when I start to utter the phrase, and in the heated moment he responds, 'I know, I know, Dad, Honor the Game.'"

Matt admits it doesn't always work, but adds that it's the best thing he's found for coaching his own kids. The groundwork must be clearly understood when parents coach their children. The emotional exchanges between parent-coach and child-athlete must be subdued. Each player on the team must be treated as an equal. Discipline, playing time, praise, and reprimands must be delivered without regard to ability or family ties.

⇨ *Let kids be kids!*

Yes, we want our kids to have fun, and we want them to feel they belong. So, all you parents and coaches remember this important concept:

If a child thinks he did okay, he's going to have fun. In the end, this might be better than winning a trophy.

"Show Me the Money," Billy's Story

Billy was only 7 when his parents took him to the local gym to join the junior basketball league. Despite his young age, his parents knew he would be the best athlete on the team. Before the season was 6 weeks old, sure enough, Billy had distinguished himself. The other parents watched in amazement as the ball was passed to Billy. This little kid had remarkable coordination and speed.

But the coaches weren't happy. It looked as if Billy's only objective was to score for himself, not the team. One said, "Billy is playing only for himself. What's going on here?"

"I don't know," the other coach admitted.

A few weeks later, the coaches had their first clue, when Billy's dad called one of the team coaches and said, "My son is not getting the ball passed to him often enough."

"We try to give every child a chance," the coach explained. "That's what our league is about . . . ."

Billy's father interrupted. "You don't understand. Billy is an unbelievable point guard, and you're not playing him enough."

"But the overall purpose of the league is . . . ." the coach continued, but Billy's father wasn't listening. He wanted more action for his son, the point guard.

Frustrated, the coach called the team's other coach and repeated Billy's father's message.

The second coach exploded. "Point guard? He can't differentiate a point guard from a box of Goobers. 'Point guard' is father talk, not kid talk. Something's going on here that we don't know about."

A week later, the coaches did some snooping on their own and learned that Billy's dad paid him 25 cents for every basket that he made. The coaches called a parents' meeting, and at the meeting they announced that any player who was rewarded individually by a parent for his performance would be banned from the team.

It took less than a month for Billy to become a team player. Oh, and by the way, Billy was *seven* years old at the time.

"My Kid Hates Sports," Craig's Story

Craig was one of those kids whose father couldn't figure out why his son hated team sports. Craig's dad is a friend of mine, and he called and said, "Craig hates basketball and his coach, and he doesn't want to play. But I think he's a boy who needs team sports. Would you take him on one of your teams?"

Of course I agreed. I figured the kid was probably not the greatest, but that didn't mean he couldn't be on a team. So, Craig came to practice. After observing him, I didn't think it likely that he would ever be a high-scoring player. I knew that if I put him in a position where all eyes would be focused on his scoring, he'd hate the game, himself, his parents, and all the other kids. He'd also hate the coach, and I wasn't going to let that happen.

So, I put on my thinking cap and realized how Craig could excel. I also knew exactly how he could contribute and help my team win.

"Okay, Craig, see this back line? You're going to stand here with your foot on the line, and when anyone on the other team comes toward you and tries to run past you, just keep your foot on that line. The opposing player will surely run 'out of bounds.'"

I looked straight into Craig's eyes after this statement and firmly shouted, "Got it?" Craig got it. I watched him during the game, and he did just what I had asked him to do. He paid attention and was alert throughout. At the end of the game, which our team won by 11 points, I gathered the guys together and said, "Okay, who was the star of this game?" One kid pointed to the fellow who scored 10 points; another pointed to the one who scored 8. But I said, "No. The star of the game was Craig. He scored 12 points."

"No, he didn't," said one of the kids.

"Yes, he did," I answered.

Another kid said, "Coach, Craig didn't even take a shot."

I knew I had the attention of the entire team. "Listen guys. By maintaining his position under the basket and playing good defense, Craig prevented six baskets from being scored against us, and those 12 points were the difference between us winning and losing."

The kids acted as if they'd just learned something incredible, something they'd never even considered. They all looked at Craig and began high-fiving him. "Way to go, Craig!" one shouted, "Craig, you got us the win!" another yelled. After the game, Craig went home with a gleaming smile on his face. That night, Craig's father called. "I don't know what happened," he said, "but now my kid loves basketball and can't wait for the next game."

Perhaps your kid is truly a talented player. You might even be realistic enough to know that his present talent level might never blossom into what you hope it might, but right now you think he needs a league that offers better competition. I am totally supportive. There are many options for the younger athlete who is inherently a gifted athlete, much as the gifted student should be placed in advanced academic tracks such as honors or AP programs. Travel Teams and AAU programs are wonderful options for such athletes. The major drawback is *commitment*. These programs often place extremely high and often unrealistic demands on both the athlete and parents. If you are able to work with this type of hectic schedule, these programs can be very good. However, young athletes should not focus on only one sport, year round. Many travel programs, and travel coaches in particular, impose unrealistic demands and require year-round commitment. This should be a serious consideration in your decision.

Reading the Coach's E-mail

Q: Why doesn't my kid play more? You're the coach of a Little League team, and your kid plays more than mine. Why?

A: The rules change in the major's division of Little League. We try to give younger athletes equal opportunities to bat. But, as kids get older, they have to understand that coaches begin to look for special qualities in their players: talent and attitude. Adults who coach older kids have a responsibility to do more than just rotate playing opportunities. It's also the coach's responsibility to reward outstanding talent and attitude. This is a part of the life lessons that we all try to teach and, of course, the rules don't change for the coach's son. I know it's my job to make sure *all* the kids on my teams earn their playing time.

Q: Can you teach my son some of the cool plays we see basketball players do on televised games?

A: Of course not. As a coach, it's my job to reel in young athletes and keep them from harm by teaching the fundamentals of the game, the essentials of early skill development, and an appreciation for their own limitations. I teach for success—not coach for failure.

Q: I've agreed to coach my daughter's baseball team (the kids are under the age of 10), and for the first session I'd like to emphasize the essentials of fair play. Do you have any suggestions for talking to them?

A: First, promise them fun. This, more than anything else, will get their attention. Begin by playing with them. It can be a relay—anything simple–so you can get a sense of their willingness to play together cooperatively and have a good time.

As you watch them, you'll get an idea of which kids are considerate of others. Move them around gently so that everyone plays a fair amount. Don't put too much pressure on the kids who have less talent. The better players won't mind if they don't play as much, but you'll lose less talented kids if they don't play at all.

Over time, you'll continue to study them and their talents, and learn to position them so they can be successful. It is certainly a coach's goal to afford every child an opportunity to try every position. However, as the coach, you must assure safety and success for each player. A child should not be placed at a position where she is doomed to fail or—worse yet, likely to be injured.

Q: My son is on a Little League team, and I think he is having trouble seeing balls in the outfield. When should his eyes be examined?

A: Immediately! A child's first visual examination should take place before the age of 6 months, and again at 3 and at 5 years. Your school-age child should be evaluated every 2 years and/or at the first sign of any problems.

Conclusion

Parents are highly qualified to be coaches, but the job comes with responsibilities and the need to understand what's involved. In coaching, parents need to be supportive teachers with reasonable expectations.

chapter 6

keeping kids safe while they have fun

A GUIDE TO COMMON INJURIES AND HOW TO MANAGE THEM

Dr. Rob, how can we keep our kids safe and still let them have fun?

Use your common sense! Don't overplay the sniffles or ignore possible injuries. When in doubt, remember guys like me. We don't mind answering your questions, and we'd rather X-ray a kid than let him play untreated. If your child is hurt or feeling sick, it's your job to keep him at home. Honestly, the game is not the most important thing in the world, but your child's health *is*.

Let me tell you a few stories so you'll understand what I mean:

Ritchie was a star pitcher on one of my Little League teams. The kid was a coach's dream. Not only was he a talented athlete, he was also a true team player who came equipped with one of the essentials: supportive and understanding parents. They were there the day Ritchie slid into second and got up holding his elbow and moaning.

As a doctor and a coach, I immediately took him out of the game. I could see that his pain was severe, and his elbow was already inflamed and red. My field-side exam did not reveal any serious injury, but Ritchie didn't believe me. He was hurting. His parents asked what they should do.

"Rest," I said. "Let's see how he feels tomorrow. If need be, I'll examine him again, and I might need to order X-rays." I told them it was possible that Ritchie might be out for several weeks. Before they left the field, I looked carefully at his elbow and added, "Absolutely no pitching or throwing until your elbow is pain-free."

The next week Ritchie's dad called and said, "What did you mean by 'no throwing'?"

I replied, "I meant that Ritchie should not pick up a ball until we are sure he is healed and there is no significant injury."

Two weeks later, Ritchie's dad was on the phone again. "Well, if he feels better by 3 weeks, can he throw a short distance?'

"No! No pitching until he is medically cleared."

Three weeks after the injury, Ritchie's dad came to the field with him. "Rob, this is amazing. I can tap his elbow and he doesn't feel any pain."

"Come here, Ritchie," I said. When I tapped his elbow in the "right" spot, he yelled "oww."

The next day I had Ritchie come in for an X-ray and an MRI (magnetic resonance imaging) of his elbow. (An MRI is a very detailed picture of the muscles, bones, nerves, and organs.) I showed Ritchie's dad the areas of bone irritation and ligament damage on the images. Finally, Ritchie's dad heard me. I didn't need the X-ray and MRI to make the diagnosis, but his parents did.

I have learned time and time again that medical concerns are not always in concert with coaching concerns. One-third of all kids who pitch in Little League wind up with shoulder and/or elbow pain in later life. The real risk is that the injuries will affect the growing part of the bone and do permanent damage that will become the source of lifelong pain.

⇨ *Is any game worth a lifetime of pain?*
Let me answer that for you: "NO!"

Of course, it isn't just eager parents and players who overlook the doctor's advice. Managers and other coaches can also cause trouble:

Cory was one of the best players I've ever seen, a true all-star pitcher and catcher. He cut his leg in a household accident and required 15 stitches.

Two days later, the manager of his team, who was getting the team ready to play in the championship series, called me and said, "Can Cory play if he has a compress on his leg and we get a runner for the bases for him?"

"No," I said firmly.

"But I spoke with his mother, and she said it would be okay," he assured me.

"NO!" I repeated.

The next day, I went to the baseball game, and there was Cory on the field. "The show must go on," and "Get out there and play for our team no matter how you feel," are adult concepts. With his leg wrapped and bandaged like a mummy, Cory hobbled about on the field, but fortunately he never reached first base that night. Children need time, space, and permission to heal after each of life's hurts in order to grow up healthy.

"Let kids be kids" also means "Let kids be *healthy* kids."

Better Safe than Sorry

Every organized sports league has—or should have—a safety committee to supervise the safety of the playing environment and the players. The responsibilities of the safety committee should be twofold: to obtain medical clearance from the child's physician assuring that the child is medically able to play and detailing any limitations; and the distribution and collection of a medical information form from each player. The medical form should contain the following information:

- The child's name, address, and relevant phone numbers
- The parents' work and cell phone numbers
- Social Security number (for emergency use if transportation to a hospital is necessary)
- Physician's name and phone numbers
- Height and weight of the player, because sometimes emergency medicines are given in dosages according to the size of the child
- Medical history (special conditions and childhood illnesses)
- Allergies (medical, food, and environmental)
- Current medications being taken by the child
- Preferred hospital

Kids' Health Problems

The most common ailments among kids who go out for sports are seasonal allergies and asthma. It's mandatory for parents to identify children with these problems so that the coach can be certain that a parent or caregiver for the child is

Water Safety

I am always concerned when kids are near water. If there is a pool, pond, or lake nearby, there can never be too many parents on watchful duty.

I once saw a 2-year-old crawl on the tarp of a covered pool: she had to be lured back to safety because the tarp was too fragile to hold the weight of an adult rescuer.

Big floats in pools are also a safety hazard. While at a pool party with adults, we learned that a child was stuck in the middle of a float. A father, fully dressed, jumped into the pool and brought the child out.

Another time, again while the parents were present but not watching, a 2-year-old jumped into the pool and was rescued—fortunately—by someone who just happened to see him

always present at practice sessions and games with *all* the proper medications. If someone cannot be there, it's essential that the parent speaks with the coach and is sure the coach is aware of the child's medical conditions and how to intervene should an emergency arise.

Some of the common medications coaches have become familiar with are: eye drops, saline solution, Benadryl®, and asthma inhalers for acute flare-ups. All of the necessary medications should be available a few feet from the field, in the possession of an adult. Should the adult need to leave, the medication should be given to the coach or the child to be used in case of an emergency.

An EpiPen® is often used for children with significant allergies. This device looks very much like a ballpoint pen, but it's filled with medication that helps to thwart an allergic reaction. Most people who carry an EpiPen® are familiar with how to administer the medication by giving an injection with it. If you are a coach, and one of your athletes carries an EpiPen®, I urge you to develop a strategy with the parents for when they are not around, in case the EpiPen® is needed to treat an allergic reaction.

Common Injuries

Despite precautions and safety warnings, injuries do occur in young athletes. It's important for parents to recognize and treat them as required.

Sprains and Strains

Luckily, the injuries sustained by most kids heal with time, because the most common ones are sprains (damage to a ligament) and strains (damage to a muscle or tendon). The most common of these is the "twisted" ankle. *Symptoms* of an ankle injury include pain (commonly felt along the outer side of the ankle), mild swelling, and discoloration of the skin.

It can take 3–6 weeks for proper healing of a sprain or strain. A general guideline is that if the child can walk on the sprained or strained area, the injury is probably not too serious.

Treatment sometimes confuses parents. Heat or ice? Ice is recommended for an acute sprain or strain, and moist heat is the treatment of choice after a few days, when the swelling has gone down. The acronym **RICE** is the sequence for treatment after an injury:

- R: Rest
- I: Ice
- C: Compression
- E: Elevation

Rest is needed only until the child can move on his own.

Ice should be wrapped in a towel and applied to the area 5 minutes on, 5 minutes off, 3–4 times a day for a minimum of 45 minutes per day.

Compression helps reduce swelling and is used for the first few days after an injury. Be sure the wrap is not applied too tightly, which might damage nerves under the skin and/or reduce blood flow to the area and produce tissue damage.

Elevation helps to reduce swelling. Elevate the injured arm or leg above the level of the heart. This allows the accumulated fluid from the swelling to drain toward the heart.

Contact your physician if the injured area does not improve after several days, or if there is any loss of strength or sensation. Also, be sure to talk to your doctor before giving your child any medications, because many children are sensitive to them.

Overuse Injuries

Many children's injuries are the result of direct blows, such as falling from a bicycle; other injuries are caused indirectly—for example, a twisted knee caused by running on a soccer field. But, by far, the most common injury is *overuse*.

What is overuse? Exactly what it says—doing too *much,* too *fast,* too *often*. An overuse injury is the body's normal reaction to abnormal stress, and it can take one of three forms: tendonitis, stress fractures, and shin splints.

Tendonitis

Tendonitis is a condition that commonly results from overuse. This term relates to inflammation of a tendon, the part of the muscle that attaches it to bone. Common areas of injury are the ankle (Achilles tendonitis), sole of the foot (plantar fasciitis), knee (patellar tendonitis), and shoulder (rotator cuff strain). (For more information on rotator cuff injuries, see the section that follows on shoulder injuries). Usually, tendons are very strong and resilient. However, repeated stress can cause them to become inflamed.

Symptoms of tendonitis include localized pain, soreness, and the inability to effectively use the affected limb or body part. This type of injury takes time to heal in children and adults. However, adult recovery takes 4–6 weeks, but children often heal in 3–4 weeks. Common types of tendonitis include:

- *Achilles tendonitis* can occur in people who run a lot, and is characterized by pain in the lower leg. A child with this type of tendonitis might complain of extreme tenderness at the back part of the heel. This might reflect an injury known as *Sever's apophysitis*. This condition is most common during the early teen years. It's caused by irritation where the Achilles tendon attaches to the heel bone (calcaneus). It usually subsides on its own, but placing a gel cushion in the heel area of the shoe often helps to reduce the discomfort.

- *Plantar fasciitis* is a common complaint among children. It starts with pain along the sole of the foot and near the heel, with discomfort when the child walks or runs. Also, the pain can be worse the first thing in the morning, with the first few steps she takes after getting out of bed. This injury requires rest, physical therapy, and possibly a shoe insert (orthotic) if your child's foot tends to have arches that fall as she walks. Sometimes, even a special brace is utilized (a foot splint).

- *Patellar tendonitis* has become common in young kids. With this condition, the pain is localized directly below the kneecap and is almost always the result of an overuse injury. If the pain is noted slightly lower and over a little "bump" on the top of the shinbone, it might indicate a condition called *Osgood-Schlatter*, an injury to an area of growing bone. Many kids find playing sports very difficult when this injury occurs. It's helpful to rest, and then slowly strengthen the muscles of the lower limb.

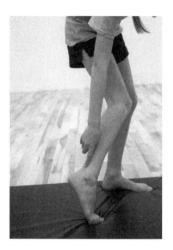 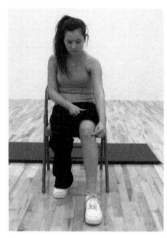

Left: Achilles tendonities
Right: Patellar tendonitis

Treatment for all of these overuse injuries involves similar strategies. In addition to resting the affected area, including icing through a towel (5 minutes on, 5 minutes off for at least 45 minutes per day), and gentle stretching, a program of strengthening should begin once improvement is noted. As an added precaution, make sure that your child does a 5-minute warm-up before exercising. Stretching is recommended for every growing child in order to stretch the tissues and keep them as pliable as possible. When stretching, *never* bounce the area being stretched. To relax the muscle, you might want to apply a warm towel for 5 minutes before stretching.

Stress Fracture

This term does not refer to the typical broken bone or fracture, but to a disruption of a portion of a bone. Imagine a dry tree branch; the branch will likely snap in half if you bend it. On the other hand, a very wet tree branch might fold if you bend it, but it probably will not snap in half—the integrity of the branch is disrupted but it remains whole. A stress fracture is similar. It develops over time, causing localized pain and increased discomfort with weight-bearing pressure on the affected bone. It might take 2 weeks from the time of injury for a stress fracture to appear on an X-ray. However, two other diagnostic tools may expedite identification of a stress fracture: a *bone scan* and magnetic resonance imaging (MRI).

A bone scan involves taking a picture of the affected body part with a special camera (much like a Geiger counter) that can often identify the area of bone with the stress fracture. This procedure involves injecting a radioactive dye into a vein. The dye circulates through the blood system and tends to be attracted to areas of the damaged bone. When the picture is taken with the special camera, the stress fracture appears as a "dark" area. The MRI is quite different. With this machine, another type picture is taken, but no injection is needed. Rather, the patient is placed into a special machine that takes a very detailed picture of the involved area that can identify subtle changes of bone, such as a stress fracture.

Treatment is rest, of course, and the child should refrain from weight-bearing sports for 6–8 weeks. Non–weight bearing activities such as swimming are recommended. If the stress fracture recurs, further diagnostic evaluations will be needed. The first question that will be asked is whether the child reduced weight-bearing stress so that healing could take place. The next will be to find out whether the child's diet contains adequate calcium and vitamin D. Any deficiency can be reversed by drinking 2–3 glasses of milk each day.

Another possible cause for recurrent stress fractures is *biomechanical error*, meaning that the foot does not absorb the stress load of the child's body weight when it strikes the ground. The most effective way to reduce this load is by limiting the injured area contacting the ground, most often by using a cane or crutches to reduce stress to the limb.

Medical causes might be present as well, such as metabolic disorders that can lead to stress fractures. Your physician might need to perform additional blood tests, and possibly other tests, to help determine the cause. Metabolic disorders such as hormonal imbalances can lead to stress fractures resulting from altered calcium and phosphorous levels.

Shin Splints

Shin splints are caused by inflammation of the tendons of the lower leg where they attach to the shin. The treatment is the same as that for tendonitis.

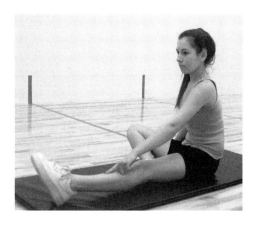

Overuse injuries are a nuisance. I sometimes think of them as "abuse" injuries. Kids who play on multiple teams because of their involvement in several leagues at the same time are most likely to develop this type of problem. Repetitive strain injuries lead to overuse injuries, and overuse injuries lead to "burnout." When kids "burnout," they are often done playing sports, *any* sport.

⇨ *Kids need to rest when they are injured!*

Although proper stretching and strengthening techniques can help, parents, coaches, and friends need to pay attention when signs of injury are present. Some kids will try to "cover up" an injury so they don't miss playing time; others will magnify the complaint for reasons ranging from not wanting to play to seeking added attention. The majority of kids, however, will show subtle signs that coaches and adults need to be aware of. These signs range from a young athlete with a shoulder injury who suddenly has a decrease in his pitch velocity, to the young track star who now walks with an obvious yet sometimes subtle limp.

Elbow Injuries

"Little League elbow" is a common injury. With this condition, the pain first appears on the inner aspect of the elbow (the same side as your pinky). It is usually the result of throwing too much, but it can sometimes—only sometimes— be related to improper throwing mechanics. The elbow area is vulnerable in young children, and the biggest culprit for injury is overuse, with resulting damage to the supporting structures of the elbow.

A child's ligaments are strong, and the injury might be a simple sprain. The

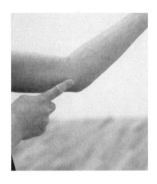

ligament involved (the ulnar collateral ligament) extends from the lower part of the arm to the upper part of the forearm and travels right across the elbow. When it's severely pulled or stretched, the ligament can exert pressure on the elbow bone at the point where it's attached. The top layer of this bone is called the *epicondyle*—and because ligaments in kids are very strong, the tension of the ligament might actually pull off and detach part of the elbow bone. When the ligament is injured and the bone is involved, it's called *medial epicondylitis, traction apophysitis*, or—in simple terms—*Little League elbow.*

Symptoms are soreness in the region of the "funny bone," possibly swelling, and mild redness. Pain will increase when the child throws. The parents and coach need to share information about the child's symptoms because, if left untreated, this injury can result in a lifelong problem. It might even affect the growth of the bone in that region, because this area contains a *growth plate*, an area from which bones elongate as the child grows.

Treatment involves rest and *absolutely no throwing* until the region is pain-free. Ice the area through a towel (5 minutes on, 5 minutes off) for at least 45 minutes a day. If you're lucky, it will only take 2–3 weeks to heal, although it might take as long as several months. If pain persists for more than 2 weeks, be sure to take the child to the doctor to assess the problem.

Shoulder Injuries

A brief course in anatomy will help parents to better understand these injuries. The shoulder (glenohumeral) joint is where the arm (humerus bone) and the wing bone/shoulder blade (scapula) meet.

The shoulder joint is lined with a thin rim of cartilage called the *labrum,* which serves to cushion the area. The collar bone (clavicle) is also part of the shoulder joint. It runs from the breastbone to the wing bone and attaches to it in an area called the *acromioclavicular(AC) joint.*

The humerus (arm bone) actually floats alongside the scapula, and is held there by ligaments (structures that hold bones together) and muscles (structures that move joints). The best known of these muscles are those that make up the *rotator cuff.* Another muscle of note is the *biceps*, which runs from the elbow to the wing bone. This muscle permits us to bend the elbow. With this quick background, let's talk about the shoulder injuries that can occur in child athletes.

Rotator Cuff Injury

The main *symptom* is weakness, which is especially noticeable when the arm is outstretched. You might notice the child just doesn't throw as hard as he used

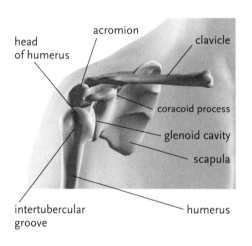

head of humerus
acromion
clavicle
coracoid process
glenoid cavity
scapula
intertubercular groove
humerus

to. There can be a "dead-arm" feeling— the arm just doesn't feel right. If a child complains of these symptoms, seek medical help *immediately.* Rotator cuff injuries most often involve a strain, not an actual tear, and healing is possible without surgery. *Treatment* requires physical therapy 2–3 times a week for a time period that can range anywhere from 2 weeks to 4 months. *No overhead throwing is permitted until all symptoms have disappeared.* Medications are rarely needed, and icing the shoulder often helps.

Bursitis

This is an inflammation of the tissues around the shoulder, and it's often associated with rotator cuff injuries. The primary *symptom* is pain, particularly when the arm is brought across the chest. *Treatment* consists of rest, ice, and medications as prescribed. In rare cases, a cortisone injection can be considered, but this is very rarely used in kids.

Remember, please, that medical cortisone is not the same as the anabolic steroids taken for performance enhancement, the kind we deplore among athletes. Medical cortisone has different properties, and can be beneficial when prescribed and administered by a physician. Still, there is no medicine without potential downsides. Cortisone should be used only for children with significant pain and disability—and only after consultation with the child's pediatrician and a sports care physician.

Acromioclavicular Joint Injury

An injury to the AC joint is usually caused by direct trauma such as a fall and, if the fall is severe, the joint might be dislocated. *Treatment* is rest, and a sling can provide comfort. As the pain subsides, let your child use the arm. This condition rarely requires surgery.

Head injuries

The most common head injuries are the most frightening: concussion or brain injury. Less than 10 percent of concussions result in loss of consciousness, so concussion is not always correctly diagnosed on the playing field. The symptoms are dizziness, nausea, headache, altered vision, a vacant stare, confusion, altered equilibrium, and even personality and behavior changes.

A concussion is always a possibility if your child is playing an *at-risk* sport such as ice hockey, wrestling, football, gymnastics, lacrosse, or soccer. Often, a concussion can be avoided if the child uses the appropriate safety equipment, primarily a helmet. The rule is to *always* seek medical help, and do your best to remain calm. Take the child to the doctor, no matter how mild the injury might seem. Following any head injury, parents should watch for signs of fatigue, irritability, headaches, equilibrium changes, and difficulty in concentrating.

If your child has a concussion, the first thing she'll want to know is when she can return to playing. Many schools of thought are related to this evolving field of medicine. A *mild concussion* is defined as one that involves no loss of consciousness and no loss of memory. If your child's concussion symptoms last less than 15 minutes, no loss of consciousness occurs, and the child can remember what happened right before and right after the injury, she can return to the playing field after 2 weeks.

Conclusion

Using common sense is the most important ingredient for ensuring your kids are safe and have fun when they play, exercise, and join in team sports. When in doubt, always take the child to his doctor to be evaluated for an injury or medical condition.

chapter 7

a few very important words about alcohol, drugs, and other threats to the safety of kids

Okay, Dr. Rob. I get it about sprains, strains, and pains but this isn't your grandma's world. Talk to us about how steroids, alcohol, drugs, and tobacco threaten our children

In December of 2007, a startling report of an investigation lead by former Senate Majority Leader George Mitchell rocked the sports world. After a 21-month investigation, this 409-page report revealed allegations that approximately 80 former and current major league players illegally used performance-enhancing substances. While the world of professional sports fans was seemingly taken aback by this revelation, I was appalled. I certainly understand the ramifications for major league baseball, and I certainly have concerns for the well-being of the many professional athletes who haphazardly choose such a wrong path. However, my fear lies in the impression this report makes on the 60 million young minds who read, view, and hear all the hype surrounding the use of such illicit substances.

My true concern is best explained by the old word game, "Association." You remember that game: I say a word and you say the first thing that pops into your mind. Well, try this game with your 11-year-old budding superstar. Mention Barry Bonds and he'll be thinking "Homeruns-Steroids." Now mention Roger Clemens, and once again, he will associate pitching success with steroids. And what do you think runs through his mind next? That's right—he's now wondering, "Hey, how can I get some of those steroids?" If nothing else, the Mitchell Report is a wake-up call to every parent, guardian, and coach of our future generations. Each of us needs to sit down with our loved ones and discuss this issue. Not only is the use of performance-enhancing substances a bad philosophical choice, it is a bad medical choice. The lure is very strong, but we must be stronger. Punishment is certainly a deterrent but education and instilling common sense may be the best antidote.

No matter how much you encourage your kids to exercise, play team sports, and eat healthy food, your efforts can be derailed by uncontrolled factors in their environment. All of your carefully laid plans for your kids can be ruined by the "big four"—steroids, alcohol, drugs, and tobacco. Children are exposed to these temptations every day on the street and at school.

Although you might think these threats won't affect *your* kids, the use of illicit substances is being seen at younger and younger ages. When you were in middle school, it was very unlikely that 20 percent of your peers were consuming alcohol on a regular basis. Guess what? Twenty percent of your child's middle school classmates *are drinking*. Let me take this one step further, but brace yourself, because the statistics aren't pretty. According to the Center for Addiction and Substance Abuse (CASA) and the 2007 National Survey of American Attitudes on Substance Abuse XII, 80 percent of high school students and 44 percent of middle grade students observe drugs being used, kept, and sold by their classmates. They also routinely see other students drunk and/or high on school grounds. Stated simply, these substances have infiltrated our school systems and are reaching children at alarmingly earlier ages.

The social challenges are mounting, and the detective work that is needed must be started early. Smart parents already recognize the scariest part of parenting—keeping kids from succumbing to pressure from their peers and experimenting with dangerous substances.

Alcohol

Parents can control the use of alcohol. I'm shocked at the number of parents who don't realize the enormity of this problem, and even more shocked by those who think teen, or even preteen, drinking is just fine as long as it's done at home under parental supervision. If I was broadcasting my 1050 ESPN radio show to you right now, I would repeat this ten times:

⇨ *The consumption of alcohol by underage kids is never acceptable. Period! Finis! End of discussion!*

Interesting Facts

- Underage drinking is a leading cause of death among young people, according to the American Medical Association. Further, drinking contributes substantially to motor vehicle crashes, suicide (28 percent of suicides among kids aged 9–15 are attributed to alcohol), date rape, and family/school problems.
- Eleven thousand underage kids in the United States try alcohol for the first time every day.
- Twenty percent of all middle school kids drink alcohol on a regular basis.
- Four kids die every day because of alcohol consumption.
- Alcohol is by far the most used and abused drug among America's teenagers. In a recent national survey, nearly one-third of all high school students reported "hazardous" drinking, including binge drinking, which is defined as more than five drinks in a given setting.

The most frightening aspect of underage drinking is the accessibility of alcohol in the home. Two out of three kids say it's easy to get alcohol at home without their parents' knowledge or consent. Here are a few simple, preventative things parents can do to help:

- Put a lock on the liquor cabinet.
- Don't *ever* permit liquor to be served to kids in your home. Prom Night parties are no excuse. Even if you're there to supervise, no liquor should ever be offered or served to children. Many local and state legislatures have passed laws holding parents liable for any and all injuries that result from serving alcoholic beverages to minors on their premises. The law can go so far as to include damages occurring off-premises.
- Monitor the reading and television viewing of your children, including text and advertising, and programming and commercials. The Center on Alcohol

Marketing and Youth (www.camy.org) evaluates and assesses the marketing of alcohol to young people. They have found a significant number of ads for alcohol in *Rolling Stone* (31 percent of readers are 12–20 years of age), *Vibe* (31 percent of readers in the same age group), and *The Source* (46 percent of readers are underage). On TV, alcohol ads were seen on the fifteen most popular TV teen shows, and let's not forget the danger of the Internet: 3 percent of visits to alcohol-related Web sites are made by underage kids.

How to Recognize Alcohol Poisoning

One of the most dreaded phone calls a parent can get is from someone asking them to come to the hospital because their child has alcohol poisoning, which has occurred for the obvious reason: the child consumed too much alcohol. Alcohol poisoning is an unconscious or semiconscious state that happens after a binge or high-volume drinking session. No, don't let someone sleep it off, especially a child, because you are dealing with a life-threatening illness and action is required.

The signs of alcohol poisoning include:

- Slow respiration (fewer than eight breaths a minute with significant lapses between breaths)
- Cold, clammy, skin
- Bluish hue to the skin
- Vomiting
- Seizures

If you notice any of these signs, immediate action is required:

- Call for medical help and take the child to the nearest medical facility.
- Try to keep the child awake; breathing can become a problem if he passes out as a result of the slowing of bodily functions.
- Keep the victim on his side to avoid swallowing vomit.
- Remove any sharp objects near the person, and move him away from the corner of the bed or place him on the floor to avoid injury in case of a seizure.
- Do not administer anything by mouth because of the danger of gagging and vomiting.

The Seduction of Anabolic Steroids

If your 12-year-old suddenly gains 30 pounds, his voice deepens, and he has an outbreak of acne, I caution you that this might not be a normal growth spurt but an indication that he is taking steroids.

"Hey guys, want to be the sports star of your school?"

"And you girls; do you want a body like a movie star?"

"Try steroids. They'll propel you to superstardom just like professional athletes and supermodels."

Kids seem to think that steroids mean glitz and glamour. They don't know about or understand the dangerous side effects of steroid use. So, it's up to parents to watch for the danger signs.

What can you as a parent do to prevent steroids from becoming a viable choice for the children in your care? Most importantly, don't push them beyond their natural physical talents, because it can cause them to seek steroids to get that extra performance "boost."

It's estimated that more than one million high school athletes are taking steroids. Even more alarming is the news that middle school kids are now hooked on steroids, too, and teenage girls are a fast-growing group of users.

It can take years for the side effects of steroids to manifest, but there are early danger signs that parents of both boys and girls should be aware of:

- Acne
- Bloating
- Unusual weight gain
- Clotting abnormalities
- Jaundice (which can indicate possible liver damage)
- Heart attacks
- Elevated cholesterol
- Weakened tendons
- Trembling
- Bad breath
- Behavioral changes (including agitation, depression, or irritability)

If you suspect that your child is experimenting with steroids, take her to your physician, and tell the doctor in advance that you suspect steroid use. This is a tough road for a parent to face alone, and you will need professional help.

⇨ *Anabolic steroids are not a recreational drug.*
They are potent and lethal!

Over time, anabolic steroids can cause boys to have a reduced sperm count, impotence, breast enlargement, shrinking testes, and painful urination. Girls might develop facial hair, deepened voice, breast reduction, and menstrual irregularities.

Conclusion

The information in this chapter was not written to scare you, but to warn you. You can't just be your kid's best friend; you have to also be a grown-up, with the power to make the final decisions regarding the health and welfare of the children who have been entrusted to your safekeeping.

chapter 8

meal plans and sports menus for kids who think they hate healthy foods

TONI COLARUSSO, M.S.

I don't know what to do, Dr. Rob. I've tried everything, but my kids just tune me out when I tell them to eat something because it's healthy.

Of course they do. That's the wrong way to convince them. You need a "vocabulary transfusion." Instead of asking kids to eat *healthy* food, why not talk about *power* foods? You can also relate power foods to sports. Explain to your child that the better he eats, the better his performance will be.

Adults often lay down rules that children think are too strict and uncompromising. Let's face it—kids today live in a world filled with junk food, and they love it. With this in mind, our goal must be to incorporate all the good foods we can into their diet. Most adults overlook the fact that even *talking* about the right foods can be fun.

One day, I walked into the locker room of the New York Knicks and saw Greg Brittenham, the assistant coach for strength and conditioning, blending a batch of drinks—red, blue, and yellow. "What in the world are you doing?" I asked.

"Mixing fruit drinks for the guys."

"Fruit drinks? Why?"

"Because I believe a pre-game drink is great for an extra boost of energy. I even make certain drinks for certain players."

This made me think about the teams I coach. If special drinks work for professional athletes, why not create sports diets for kids? Isn't it about time that we made healthy eating *fun* for our kids?

I went to see Toni Colarusso, a dietitian in private practice, because I consider her to be one of the best in her field. Together, Toni and I created healthy meal plans that can help kids create a lifetime of good eating habits. These plans were created specifically for kids who think they hate healthy foods, and we've geared everything to sports. What kid wouldn't be proud to be on the *baseball diet*, or tell her friends she's on the *soccer diet*?

The meal plans include a daily snack. Most of the time, these are healthy treats, but occasionally they are a bit sinful. We call these snacks *Toni's Treats*. Some kids need more than one snack per day to meet their caloric needs; others need less. As you read this chapter, you will learn how to calculate your child's specific calorie needs and be guided as to how to adjust the snacks to meet her needs

Of course, no one has to be on a sports team to follow these healthy food plans. You can mix and match meals and snacks from one meal plan to another, depending on your child's food preferences, as long as you stay within the child's caloric needs. Our sports diets were created so kids think of themselves as *conditioning for participation*—even if they're not active participants at the moment.

Before starting any healthy meal plan, Toni reminds us of some general guidelines parents should follow. First, as parents, you need to be role models and practice what you preach. If you eat healthy and regularly prepare healthy meals for the entire family, your child will eat healthy, too.

Meal plans should be well balanced. Your child needs to eat selections from all the food groups. The Food Pyramid can assist you with this. The figure opposite characterizes the essential foods a child requires to have a balanced diet (see also www.mypyramid.gov; additional food lists can be found at www.mendosa.com).

Calorie Requirements

In addition to eating from the food groups of the Food Pyramid, there are recommendations for the types of calories children generally require. The recommended percentage of calories for children from 5–12 years of age should come from the following food types:

- Carbohydrates: 55–75 percent (each gram of carbohydrate contains approximately 4 calories)
- Fats: 25–30 percent (each gram of fat contains approximately 9 calories)

- Protein: 15–20 percent (each gram of protein contains approximately 4 calories)

Protein Requirements

As a general guide, the protein requirements for children 5–12 years of age are:

- Ages 5–10: 25–30 grams per day
- Ages 11–12: 45–50 grams per day for girls, and 45–60 grams per day for boys

The total protein requirement may be summarized in grams per pound of body weight as in Table 1, and Table 2 gives the protein content of some common foods.

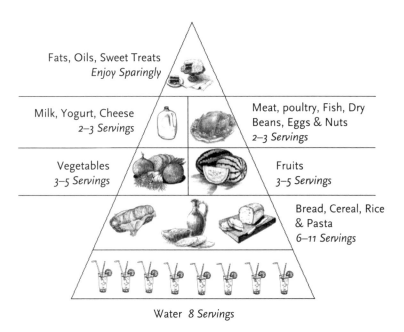

Fats, Oils, Sweet Treats
Enjoy Sparingly

Milk, Yogurt, Cheese
2–3 Servings

Meat, poultry, Fish, Dry Beans, Eggs & Nuts
2–3 Servings

Vegetables
3–5 Servings

Fruits
3–5 Servings

Bread, Cereal, Rice & Pasta
6–11 Servings

Water *8 Servings*

TABLE 1. Total Protein Requirements

Age group	Protein requirement (grams/lb body weight)
Infant	0.8
Preschool child	0.5
School child	0.5
Adult	0.3
Strength athletes	0.8
Endurance athletes	0.7

TABLE 2. Protein Content of Common Foods*

Plant-based Sources	Protein Content (grams)
Tempeh (4 oz.)	17–21
Tofu, firm (½ cup)	10
Soymilk, plain (8 oz.)	10
Soybeans, black, cooked (½ cup)	14
Soybeans, green, cooked (½ cup)	11
Peanut butter, chunky (2 Tbsp)	8
Kidney beans, cooked (½ cup)	8
Black beans, cooked (½ cup)	8
Chick-peas, cooked (½ cup)	8
Hummus (¼ cup)	5
Refried beans, cooked (½ cup)	8
Pinto beans, cooked (½ cup)	7
Lima beans, cooked (½ cup)	5

* Modified from "Your Pathway to Wellness," a program of Northwestern Health Sciences University, http://www.nwhealth.edu/healthyU/eatWell/protein3.html

Peanuts (½ cup) 19

Almonds (½ cup) 15

Pine nuts (½ cup) 15

Cashews (½ cup). 10

Sunflower seeds (½ cup). 13

Walnuts (½ cup) 10

Flax seeds, ground (2 Tbsp) 4

Wheat germ (2 Tbsp) 4

Whole-wheat bread (1 oz. slice) 3

Oatmeal, instant, cooked (1 cup) 6

Broccoli (1 cup). 5

Corn (1 cup) 5

Rice, white (1 cup) 2.5

Rice, brown (1 cup). 4.5

Pasta, cooked (1 cup) 6.5

Animal-based Sources Protein Content (grams)

Chicken, boneless, cooked (3 oz.). 27

Turkey, roasted (3 oz.) 25

Ground turkey, cooked (3 oz.) 23

Roast beef, lean, cooked (3 oz.). 24

Ground beef, lean, cooked (3 oz.). 24

Beef sirloin, cooked (3 oz.) 24

Pork, roast, trimmed (3 oz.) 25

Ham, cooked (3 oz.) 21

Tuna, canned in water (3 oz.) 23

Tuna, fresh, cooked (3 oz.) 26

Yogurt, low-fat, plain (8 oz.) 12

Frozen yogurt (½ cup) 2.5

Milk (8 oz.) 8

Cheese (1 oz.) 7

Cream cheese (2 Tbsp) 4

Egg (1 medium). .6

Egg white (1) 3.5

Egg substitute (¼ cup) 6

Cottage cheese (½ cup) 14

Cod, cooked (3 oz.) 20

Salmon (3 oz.) 22

Shrimp, boiled (3 oz.) 21

Lobster, baked or broiled (3 oz.) 17

Ice milk, soft-serve (1 cup) 10

Assuming that your school-age child has 60 minutes of active play time each day, calorie requirements vary from 1,800 to 2,600. To calculate your child's specific daily calorie needs, use the following recommendations in Table 3, devised by the Food and Nutrition Board and the National Academy of Sciences-National Research Council:

TABLE 3. Calorie Guidelines per Day

Age	Calories per Day
Girls age 4–6	1,800
Boys age 4–6	2,000
Girls age 9–13	2,200
Boys age 9–13	2,600

Group	Calories Required per Pound of Body Weight per Day
Children age 4–6 41	
Children age 7–10 32	
Boys age 11–14 25	
Girls age 11–14 21	

Additional calories should be added depending on your child's extracurricular activities.

To increase daily intake by 200 calories, add any one of the following: ¼ cup nuts, 1 slice thin-crust pizza, 2 Rice Krispies treat squares, 3 cups popcorn lightly buttered, 1 taco, 4 chicken nuggets, or 1 blueberry muffin.

For an additional 300 calories, add any one of the following: a junior cheeseburger, 6 chicken nuggets, a peanut butter and jelly sandwich, or ½ cup chili with ½ cup tortilla chips.

The number of calories for each meal plan provides you with an approximate number of calories for each day. However, as a sensible parent, you can adjust servings and add or subtract snacks if you think your child needs more or fewer calories.

The Five Food Groups

As you already know—and if you don't, your child probably does—there are five essential food groups:

- Grains
- Vegetables
- Fruits
- Dairy-Milk
- Meat/Beans

Oils are also an essential part of a healthy diet and are included below.

Because each group provides your child's growing body with different nutrients, it is important to eat from all the food groups in the recommended amounts.

Grains

This group includes foods made from wheat, rice, oats, cornmeal, barley, and other cereal grain products. Grains are divided into whole grains and refined grains. Whole grains, like oatmeal, brown rice, and whole-wheat flour contain the entire grain kernel. Refined grains, including white flour, white rice, and white bread, have been processed to remove the bran and germ of the whole grain, a process that also removes dietary fiber, iron, and many of the B vitamins. Most of these foods have had iron and B vitamins added back after processing, but not the fiber. For this reason, your child's diet and your own should include whole grains whenever possible. Grains are carbohydrates, which the body uses as its major source of energy as well as fiber, B vitamins, and iron.

Children ages 5–8 require four to five 1-ounce equivalents of grains per day. By the ages of 9–12, this increases to five to six 1-ounce equivalents per day.

Vegetables

Vegetables provide important vitamins and minerals, and they are a great source of fiber and carbohydrates for energy. Fiber is important because it helps the digestive system move things along and reinforces the habits of a lifetime of good eating.

What is a 1-ounce equivalent of grains?

- 1 slice of bread
- 1 cup of ready-to-eat cereal
- ½ cup of cooked cereal
- ½ cup of cooked rice
- ½ cup of pasta

What counts as 1 cup in the vegetable group?

- 1 cup carrot slices
- 2 cups of raw leafy vegetables (lettuce, spinach)
- 1 cup of cooked or raw broccoli (chopped or florets)
- 1 cup of vegetable juice

Children ages 5–8 require 1½ cups of vegetables per day. This increases to 2–2½ cups of vegetables per day at 9–12 years of age

Fruits

Fruits, like vegetables, provide significant amounts of vitamins and minerals, and are an important source of fiber and carbohydrates. Children ages 5–8 require 1–1½ cups of fruit per day; 1½ cups per day are needed by children ages 9–12.

Dairy

The dairy group includes milk and any food made from milk, such as yogurt and cheese. This food group is important because it provides your child with calcium

What counts as 1 cup in the fruit group?

- 1 cup of fruit or 100-percent fruit juice, or ½ cup of dried fruit

- 1 cup cut-up fruit (pineapple, melon, berries)

- 1 small size fruit, 2.5-inch in diameter (apple, banana, pear, orange)

- 1 cup of canned, cooked, or dried fruit (raisins, canned fruit cocktail)

- 1 cup of 100-percent fruit juice

What counts as a cup in the milk group?

- 1 cup of milk or yogurt (preferably low-fat or fat-free)

- 1½ ounces of hard cheese (cheddar, Swiss, preferably low-fat or fat-free)

- 2 ounces of processed cheese (American, preferably low-fat or fat-free)

- 1 cup frozen yogurt

to help keep bones strong and the protein essential for growth. Children ages 5–8 require 2 cups of dairy per day, while those ages 9–12 require 3 cups.

Meat and Beans

The meat and beans group was formerly known as the *Protein* group. It includes meat, poultry, fish, eggs, beans, peas, nuts, and seeds. These foods provide protein and essential minerals such as iron and zinc. Beans and peas are part of this group; they are also included in the vegetable group.

Children ages 5–8 require three to four 1-ounce equivalents of meat per day. By ages 9–12, their requirements increase to five to six 1-ounce equivalents.

What is a 1-ounce equivalent?

- 1 ounce of cooked lean meat, poultry, or fish (a small lean hamburger patty or a small chicken breast equals 2–3 1-ounce equivalents)
- 1 egg
- ¼ cup cooked beans
- ½ ounce of nuts (12 almonds, 7 walnuts halves, 24 pistachios)
- 1 tablespoon of peanut butter or almond butter

Oils

Our bodily function depends upon the availability of fatty acids. Some fatty acids cannot be manufactured by our own body and must be supplied from other sources. Since our body cannot manufacture them on its own, these are collectively known as *essential fatty acids* (EFAs) because they are essential in our diet. We typically consume them in food, but they also can be taken as supplements. Fatty acids play a key role in the prevention of heart disease, lowering *bad* cholesterol (LDL and VLDL), stimulating brain tissue, assisting in bone repair, and many other key bodily functions. Two specific types of fatty acids have received highlighted attention recently; *Omega-3* and *Omega-6*. Both play key roles in nutrition and are supplied by many dietary sources. Omega-3 fatty acids are commonly found in plants, nuts, and fish, including cold-water fish such as salmon, mackerel, halibut, sardines, tuna, and herring. Omega-6 fatty acids are commonly found in cooking oils, including sunflower, safflower, corn, cottonseed, and soybean oils.

While both types of fatty acids are important, recent evidence suggests that their consumption should be in a balanced ratio, with approximately equal amounts of Omega-3 to Omega-6. However, our diets contain a much higher proportion of Omega-6 fatty acids (with ratios of 20:1 or more at times), and it has been sug-

---

What counts as a teaspoon of oil?

- 1 teaspoon vegetable oil (such as canola)
- ½ medium avocado equals 3 teaspoons of oil
- 2 tablespoons of peanut butter equals 4 teaspoons of oil
- 1 ounce of sunflower seeds equals 3 teaspoons of oil

---

gested that this imbalance may lead to heart disease, asthma, depression, and certain cancers.

Unfortunately, there are no agreed-upon established guidelines for the daily consumption of fatty acids. I strongly suggest you speak with a health care professional, such as a pediatrician or registered dietician, to determine whether your children are consuming adequate amounts of essential fatty acids in their diet.

Certain fats should be avoided. One group in particular is *trans fat*. These are sometimes noted on the nutrition label as hydrogenated oils, partially hydrogenated oils, or shortening. Trans fats are produced artificially (although some do naturally occur in meat products) by converting a liquid fat such as vegetable oil into a more solid form. This solid form mimics *saturated fat.* As we know, our dietary focus should be to limit the intake of saturated fats and increase the consumption of unsaturated fats, because saturated fats are the culprit in many ailments including heart disease, by clogging the arteries.

Trans fats are commonly found in fried foods, certain cookies, crackers, doughnuts, and margarine. The reason they have been utilized in the industry is they tend to add flavor to foods and can extend the shelf life for these products.

Of particular concern for me is that children who consume trans fats at an early age are positioning themselves for the early onset of heart disease and vascular problems. Unfortunately, the burden now strongly lies on mom and dad to regulate, or preferably eliminate the consumption of trans fats in our own and our children's diets. The American Heart Association recommends limiting the amount of trans fats you eat to less than 1 percent of your total daily calories. So, if you consume 2,000 calories/day, no more than 20 of those calories should come from trans fats. That's less than 2 grams of trans fats per day. The fat in your child's diet should come from fish, nuts, and vegetable oils. These oils provide the EFAs and vitamin E your child needs. Children, as well as adults, should limit their intake of fats such as butter, stick margarine, shortening, and lard.

Children ages 5–8 require 4 teaspoons of oils or fats per day. By ages 9–12, this increases to 5–6 teaspoons.

Table 4 summarizes the daily dietary requirements from the basic food groups, modified from http://www.mypyramid.gov/pyramid/index.html.

TABLE 4. Food Group Requirements
(in Ounce Equivalents-Cups/Day)

Age	Grains Ounces/Day	Vegetables Cups/D	Fruits Cups/D	Dairy Cups/D	Meats Ounces/D	Oils Tsp/D
5–8 All	4–5	1½	1–1½	2	3–4	4
Boys 9–12	6	2½	1½	3	5	5
Girls 9–12	5	2	1½	3	5	5

Healthy Eating Habits

Healthy eating optimizes athletic ability, so here are some suggestions for your young athlete's diet before, during, and after athletics. One caution: make the food choices familiar ones. Pre- or post-game times, when your child is already stressed, are not the best times to introduce new foods.

Pre-game Eating

Emphasize carbohydrates in your meal plan for the day of a game. Aim for at least the minimum number of foods offered from the grains group in order to fuel and refuel the muscles.

Snacks that digest easily are best if your child will be exercising for less than 1 hour. Bagels, bread, crackers, and pasta are popular choices.

If the exercise will last for 60–90 minutes, choose carbohydrates such as yogurt, milk, apples, and bananas, because they will increase stamina. These foods enter the bloodstream more slowly than pure grain foods because of their protein and fiber content. When foods enter the bloodstream slowly they provide sustained energy. They should be eaten approximately 1–2 hours prior to exercising.

Limit high-fat proteins such as hamburgers, peanut butter, or cheese. The fat in these foods slows down digestion and causes sluggishness. Better choices are small amounts of low-fat protein foods such as turkey, chicken, low-fat cheese, or a glass of skim or low-fat milk.

Offer sugary foods with caution. Eating or drinking foods such as jellybeans, sports drinks, soft drinks, or honey 15–120 minutes before hard exercise can result in a drop in blood sugar, causing light-headedness and decreased energy.

Remember that digestion takes time. Allow 2–4 hours between a large meal and an athletic event. This is especially important before an intense event, during which blood flow to the stomach is decreased to 20 percent of normal because the blood is diverted instead to the working muscles.

Post-game Eating

Replenishing fluids is a top priority, especially after an intense event. The best choices are water and high glycemic index foods such as fruit juices that provide

The Glycemic Index

The glycemic index (GI) has become a very popular topic, as it relates to sports and to general health. The GI is a ranking system for foods that contain carbohydrates, including grains, fruits, and vegetables. A food is ranked based on how high the blood sugar is elevated after a particular food is eaten. It was originally created to help people with diabetes better control their blood sugar levels.

Basically, foods with a high GI (a value of 60 or above) are digested more quickly and result in a quick increase in blood sugar. Foods with a moderate GI (with values of 40–60), and those with a low GI (with values less than 40), are digested more slowly and produce a gradual increase in blood sugar level. The GI response can be influenced by many factors, including a food's fiber content, the amount eaten, added fat, and the way it is prepared.

High GI foods are best eaten during or after exercise to provide quick energy. Low to moderate GI foods are best eaten before exercise, because they provide sustained energy. Low GI foods are best eaten before long-term exercise such as running a marathon to maintain normal blood sugar levels, which might eliminate the need for eating carbohydrates during the event (see Resources section).

carbohydrates as well as vitamins and minerals, watery foods such as watermelon and grapes, and high-carbohydrate sports drinks.

High-carbohydrate foods and fluids should be consumed within 15 minutes after exercise, because this is the optimum time for the muscles and body to absorb and replace the carbohydrates used during the event.

Your child's goal for replenishing carbohydrates is 0.5 grams per pound of body weight. Let's use a 60-pound, 10-year-old as an example. This child will require: 60 × 0.5 = 30 grams of carbohydrates. Because carbohydrate-containing foods contain

4 calories per gram, multiply this number by 4 to give you the number of calories from carbohydrates your child needs for replenishment: $30 \times 4 = 120$ calories from high-carbohydrate foods.

Carbohydrate-rich foods that you can offer your child after an event include:

- 1 cup of fruit juice
- ½ bagel
- 1 cup of cereal with ½ cup skim or 1 percent fat milk
- ¼ cup of raisins

Protein supplementation is also important during the recovery phase. Excessive amounts are not necessary, but combining the high-carbohydrate foods just described with protein can be a great way to refuel a child's body after an intense event. Foods rich in carbohydrates and protein that your child can try include:

- ½ bagel with 2 slices of turkey or low-fat cheese
- 8 ounces of milk
- 8 ounces of yogurt
- a small sliced apple with 2 ounces of low-fat cheese

Electrolytes, especially sodium and potassium, also need to be replaced after an intense workout or game, because these minerals are lost through perspiration. Sport drinks are a good source for electrolyte replacement.

Sodium-rich foods include pretzels, bagels, saltine crackers, and soup. Potassium-rich foods include fruit and fruit juices, potatoes, yogurt, and milk.

By following these simple guidelines, your child will not only eat sensibly every day, but will feel good before and after every activity.

Nine Ways to Cut Calories

1. Use nonstick sprays and pans instead of oils or butter.
2. Cut the calories in fruit juices and other sweetened beverages by diluting the drink with water or club soda.
3. Snack on fresh fruit instead of high-calorie dried fruit.
4. Use fat-free or low-fat dressings on your salads.
5. Get candy *out* of the house; offer kids fruit instead.
6. Use plain or vanilla yogurt, not fruit-flavored. Add fresh fruit for a burst of color, flavor, and vitamins.

7. When serving pizza, forget about cheese and meat toppings, and go for extra sauce and vegetables.

8. Forget about bagels; a whole-wheat English muffin has far fewer calories.

9. Insist that everyone in the family eat breakfast, because people who eat breakfast consume fewer calories throughout the day than those who don't eat breakfast.

Nine Ways to Eat Healthy at a Fast Food Restaurant

1. Order the thin crust type pizza with vegetable instead of meat toppings.

2. Order chicken or fish that is broiled or grilled; never deep-fried or breaded.

3. Sandwiches should be made of lean meat, plain tuna (not mixed with mayonnaise), or low-fat cheese. Stay away from sandwiches made with croissants.

4. Order single burgers, not doubles, and hold the cheese, bacon, and sauces.

5. Never order French fries or home fries; opt for baked potatoes and use low-fat toppings such as nonfat sour cream, grated cheese, chili, and chives.

6. At the salad bar, turn your back on the prepared salads. Instead, choose greens plus vegetables and/or fruit, low-fat cottage cheese, turkey, chicken, roast beef, plain tuna; always use fat-free or low-fat dressings.

7. Order plain chicken or beef-based soups with rice or noodles, mushrooms, or lentils, and avoid cream soups.

Four Healthy Kinds of Snacks

1. *Crunchies:* Pretzels, popcorn, trail mix, granola bars, and baked chips
2. *Chewies:* Bagels, dried fruit (including raisins)
3. *Yummies:* Pudding packs, milk, yogurt, and peanut butter
4. *Juicies:* Juice packs, Jell-O packs, canned fruits, and fresh fruit (grapes, oranges)

8. Avoid the fried tortillas at Tex-Mex restaurants. Choose soft tacos or burritos with chicken, beef, and vegetables. Don't reach for the sour cream; ask for the nonfat variety or use salsa.

9. At breakfast, stick to hot or cold cereal with bananas and/or granola, skim- or low-fat milk, whole-wheat toast with preserves (not butter), plain yogurt, and poached eggs.

Power and Sports Diets

There's no doubt that one of the most challenging tasks a parent faces is meal-time.

"I hate broccoli."

"I'm not eating anything orange."

"I don't like steak."

We've heard the excuses a thousand times. No matter how many times you repeat yourself by making statements like: "It's important to eat carrots because it will help your vision," your child's response is the same, a head turn and utterance of the universal "Yuck!"

With this in mind, I set out to find a way to make kids understand the importance of consuming a healthy diet and help them understand that they need certain nutrients in order to succeed on the athletic field. I just *knew* that once they understood that athletic success hinged on dietary success, I could win them over. As a result—and with the amazing imagination and coordination provided by Toni Colarusso—we developed the Power and Sports Diets.

These food plans can be mixed and mingled, but just remember to keep the calorie count where you want it. One good way is to serve all food as close to its natural state as possible. If you do, you can teach your children to appreciate the *real* taste of food—and without preaching! If you drown food in sauces and fry it in batter, you will have only added calories that no one needs, and you will have denied your kids the pleasure of eating food the way it's meant to taste.

We have included a week's worth of menu planning for each sport. Although there is a sampling of sport-specific menus, please keep in mind that these are representative *power names*, and we have not included every sport or physical activity. The goal is to offer children a user-friendly menu that will make them want to eat healthy foods, rather than eating only out of necessity or for pleasure. Of course, the food plans are not to be used for just 1 week. They mark the beginning of a lifetime of good choices. Repeat them or play with other sports choices as you continue with a life plan for your child.

Each day's menu includes substitutions, which are other foods that might be eaten, depending on the child's preference. You also need to modify the menus from each of the food groups, depending on your child's calorie needs and her age. The grain group has the largest gap in requirements between younger (ages 4–8) and older (ages 5–12) children. Please keep this in mind when you begin reviewing the meal plans for your children. This might be the group of foods you will need to modify most.

We have tried to include fun with our healthy diet suggestions, so have a good time with meals, and try some of the recipes given in the next chapter, too. Invite your kids to cook with you. It's a good way to get your young or future athlete to try new foods, and it is another positive building block in the parent–child relationship.

Weight Control

General guidelines apply to adjusting your child's weight, especially for those who want to reduce weight. Since every child grows at a different rate, it can be difficult to determine your child's optimal current weight, and the need for either weight gain or weight loss. This is further complicated by growth spurts. If you and your family are eating healthy and exercising regularly, but you are still concerned about your child's weight (whether it is too high or too low), speak with a health professional. Your child's pediatrician or a registered dietitian can help you make the correct assessment and necessary changes in the child's diet.

The 2005 Dietary Guidelines for Americans recommendations for children state that overweight children should "reduce the rate of body weight gain while allowing growth and development." This means that the child doesn't necessarily need to lose a lot of weight in the short term, but that the diet should be adjusted so he will automatically achieve a better weight for his age by "growing into it." The Guidelines also recommend consulting a health care provider before placing a child on a weight-reduction diet. As a parent, you need to support a healthy lifestyle that includes healthy eating and regular activity.

An asterisk (*) next to a food choice means that a recipe using it can be found in Chapter 9. For calorie counts with two numbers, the first number represents the calories for the food choices in the first column and the second represents the calorie count for the food choices in the second column.

Conclusion

Children can succeed in their endeavors when they are supported by healthy food choices.

⇨ *Okay, now. Everybody into the kitchen, and let's have some fun with our kids while we help them get in shape!*

Baseball Championship Meal Plans for Kids
World Series Game—Day One

HOME-RUN BREAKFAST

STEP UP TO THE PLATE	SUBSTITUTIONS	CALORIE COUNT
8 ounces orange juice	Apple, cranberry, grapefruit	100
1–2 scrambled eggs	Boiled or sunny-side-up	100–200
1 slice whole-wheat toast	Multigrain, rye	65
8 ounces skim or 1 percent fat milk		95

GRAND-SLAM LUNCH

STEP UP TO THE PLATE	SUBSTITUTIONS	CALORIE COUNT
Turkey sandwich:		
2–3 ounces turkey	*Roast beef/low-fat bologna*	75/160/*200*
2 slices of rye bread	One roll	125
2 teaspoons low-fat mayonnaise	2 tablespoons mustard	25
1 cup baby carrots	1 cup celery sticks	25
1 cup cut-up fresh fruit	¼ wedge of melon	60

TRIPLE-PLAY DINNER

STEP UP TO THE PLATE	SUBSTITUTIONS	CALORIE COUNT
**Chicken stir-fry:	Shrimp or lean beef	
1 cup chicken and vegetables		400
½ cup rice (brown is best but white is fine)		100

* Recipe in Chapter 9

TONI'S TREATS!

1 cup skim or 1 percent fat milk. 95

1 cup low-fat ice cream 200

2 graham cracker squares or 1 ice cream cone. 50

APPROXIMATE CALORIES: 1,500 FOR THE DAY

 # World Series Game—Day Two

HOME-RUN BREAKFAST

STEP UP TO THE PLATE	SUBSTITUTIONS	CALORIE COUNT
1 cup Cheerios or corn flakes	Any non–sugar coated cereal	100
1 cup skim or 1 percent fat milk.		95
1 medium banana	½ cup raisins.	100/215

GRAND-SLAM LUNCH

STEP UP TO THE PLATE	SUBSTITUTIONS	CALORIE COUNT
Cheeseburger:		
2–3 ounces lean beef	Ground turkey.	200
1 hamburger bun	2 slices whole-wheat bread	125
1–2 slices low-fat cheese		50–80
2 teaspoons low-fat mayonnaise	2 tablespoons ketchup.	30
1 medium orange	1 cup cut-up fresh fruit	60

TRIPLE-PLAY DINNER

STEP UP TO THE PLATE	SUBSTITUTIONS	CALORIE COUNT
1 medium potato, baked	½ cup rice	145/100
2–3 ounces grilled chicken	2–3 ounces grilled pork	115
1 cup cooked string beans	1 cup broccoli	80
2 teaspoons butter or oil		70

TONI'S TREATS!

5 whole-grain crackers	1 slice whole-grain bread	65
with		
2 tablespoons peanut butter	1 ounce low-fat cheese	190/50

APPROXIMATE CALORIES: 1,400 FOR THE DAY

 ## World Series Game—Day Three

HOME-RUN BREAKFAST

STEP UP TO THE PLATE	SUBSTITUTIONS	CALORIE COUNT
8 ounces apple juice	Orange juice	100
1 toasted English muffin	2 slices whole-grain toast	130
1–2 slices low-fat cheese		50–80

GRAND-SLAM LUNCH

STEP UP TO THE PLATE	SUBSTITUTIONS	CALORIE COUNT
Hot dog (low-fat):		130
hot dog bun		125
2 tablespoons mustard	2 tablespoons ketchup	25
¼ cup sauerkraut (optional)		7

1 cup baby carrots 40

2 tablespoons low-fat dressing (for dipping). 40

1 cup Jell-O with fruit. 150

TRIPLE-PLAY DINNER

STEP UP TO THE PLATE	SUBSTITUTIONS	CALORIE COUNT
*Turkey meatloaf (2–3 ounces). 145–220		
*Macaroni and cheese (1 cup) 330		
1 cup cooked spinach (steamed). 80		
(sautéed in 1 teaspoon oil) 35		
2 tablespoons turkey gravy. 15		

TONI'S TREATS!

1 cup low-fat ice cream. 200

1 medium banana . . . . ½ cup raisins. 100/215

APPROXIMATE CALORIES: 1,600 FOR THE DAY

World Series Game—Day Four

HOME-RUN BREAKFAST

STEP UP TO THE PLATE	SUBSTITUTIONS	CALORIE COUNT
1 cup cut-up fruit 60		
½ bagel	2 slices whole-wheat toast.	.125
2 tablespoons peanut butter . .	2 tablespoons low-fat cream cheese . .	.190/70

*Recipe in Chapter 9

GRAND-SLAM LUNCH

STEP UP TO THE PLATE	SUBSTITUTIONS	CALORIE COUNT
Grilled cheese sandwich:		
2 slices whole-wheat bread		125
2–3 ounces any low-fat cheese		125
2 slices tomato		10
2 teaspoons butter or margarine for grilling		70
1 cup celery sticks	1 cup cucumber slices	15

TRIPLE-PLAY DINNER

STEP UP TO THE PLATE	SUBSTITUTIONS	CALORIE COUNT
Beef and vegetable stew (1 cup	Chicken stew	200/175
½ cup rice	½ cup couscous	100
1 cup salad–mixed greens		10
2 tablespoons low-fat dressing		40

TONI'S TREATS!

½ cup cereal	2 chocolate chip cookies	50/130
1 cup skim or 1 percent fat milk		85–100
¼ cup raisins	½ cup cut-up berries	110/40

APPROXIMATE CALORIES: 1,400 FOR THE DAY

World Series Game—Day Five

HOME-RUN BREAKFAST

STEP UP TO THE PLATE	SUBSTITUTIONS	CALORIE COUNT
2 waffles (multigrain preferred)		195
1 cup strawberries	Any fresh fruit	60
1/4 cup syrup	4 tablespoons low sugar preserves	210/100
(100 for reduced calorie syrup)		
1 cup skim or 1 percent fat milk		95

GRAND-SLAM LUNCH

STEP UP TO THE PLATE	SUBSTITUTIONS	CALORIE COUNT
10 whole-grain crackers	2 slices whole-grain bread	125
2 ounces turkey	2 ounces low-fat cheese	75/100
1 cup tomato slices	1 cup tomato juice	30
2 teaspoons low-fat mayonnaise	2 tablespoons mustard	25

TRIPLE-PLAY DINNER

STEP UP TO THE PLATE	SUBSTITUTIONS	CALORIE COUNT
*Chicken fingers (2–3 oven-fried)		185
*Oven-fried sweet potato	1 medium baked potato	350/145
1 cup cooked broccoli	1 cup string beans	80
steamed or sautéed in 1 teaspoon butter or olive oil		35
1 small apple	Orange or peach	60

TONI'S TREATS!

1 cup low-fat ice cream . . . . . . 1 cup low-fat yogurt 200

1 small banana . . . . 1 cup cherries 85

APPROXIMATE CALORIES: 1,600 FOR THE DAY

⚾ World Series Game—Day Six

HOME-RUN BREAKFAST

STEP UP TO THE PLATE	SUBSTITUTIONS	CALORIE COUNT
1 cup corn flakes	Any non–sugar coated cereal	.100
1 cup skim or 1 percent fat milk		.95
1 large peach	Nectarine or banana	.80

GRAND-SLAM LUNCH

STEP UP TO THE PLATE	SUBSTITUTIONS	CALORIE COUNT
Tuna salad sandwich:		
2–3 ounces tuna in water . .	Chicken	.110
5 whole-grain crackers	1 small pita bread	.70
2 tablespoons low-fat mayonnaise		.75
½ cup tomato slices		.20
½ cup shredded lettuce		.5

TRIPLE-PLAY DINNER

STEP UP TO THE PLATE	SUBSTITUTIONS	CALORIE COUNT
Thin-crust pizza with veggie topping (1 slice)		.195

2 cups salad . . . . Cucumber slices, ...80
                                       tomato slices, carrots

2 tablespoons low-fat dressing 40

1 cup cut-up fruit 60

1 cup low-fat yogurt . . . . 1 cup skim or 1 percent fat milk 200/95

Toni's Treats!

½ cup bite-sized pretzels . . . . . 1 small pita bread 75

2 tablespoons peanut butter . . 2 tablespoons hummus 190/50

APPROXIMATE CALORIES: 1,200 FOR THE DAY

World Series Game—Day Seven

Home-run Breakfast

STEP UP TO THE PLATE	SUBSTITUTIONS	CALORIE COUNT
1 or 2 eggs 100–200		
2 strips bacon	2 sausage links 50/150	
2 slices rye toast	Whole-wheat or multigrain 125	
2 teaspoons butter	2 tablespoons low-fat cream cheese . .70	
8 ounces orange juice	Apple, cranberry, grapefruit 100	

Grand-slam Lunch

STEP UP TO THE PLATE	SUBSTITUTIONS	CALORIE COUNT
Bologna sandwich:		
2–3 ounces low-fat bologna .	Roast beef/turkey 200/160/75	
2 slices multigrain bread . . .	Whole-wheat or rye 125	

2 teaspoons low-fat . . . . 2 tablespoons mustard 25
mayonnaise

1 cup celery sticks. . . . . 1 cup cucumber slices. 15

TRIPLE-PLAY DINNER

STEP UP TO THE PLATE	SUBSTITUTIONS	CALORIE COUNT
Tacos:		
1 taco shell.	1 tortilla.	.70
2–3 ounces ground beef. . . .	Ground turkey.	.150–200
1–2 ounces low-fat cheese		.50–80
½ cup shredded lettuce		.5
½ cup cubed tomato		.20

TONI'S TREATS!

1 cup low-fat yogurt . . . . 1 cup low-fat ice cream. 200

1 cup cut-up fruit . . . . 1 small banana 75

APPROXIMATE CALORIES: 1,500 FOR THE DAY

Basketball Championship Meal Plans for Kids
NBA Finals Game—Day One

BASKET BREAKFAST

JUMPBALL	SUBSTITUTIONS	CALORIE COUNT
1 medium banana	8 ounces orange juice	100
1 cup Cheerios	Any non-frosted cereal	100
1 cup skim / 1 percent fat milk	8 ounces low-fat yogurt	95/200

FAST-BREAK LUNCH

JUMPBALL	SUBSTITUTIONS	CALORIE COUNT
Tuna salad sandwich:		
2–3 ounces tuna (canned in water)	2–3 ounces chicken	110
1 tablespoons low-fat mayonnaise	2 tablespoons mustard	40/20
1 medium tomato, sliced		30
½ cup shredded lettuce		5
1 whole-grain roll	2 slices rye bread	125

NOTHIN'-BUT-NET DINNER

JUMPBALL	SUBSTITUTIONS	CALORIE COUNT
Baked chicken (3 ounces) (marinated in Italian dressing 20 minutes before baking)		110
Spaghetti marinara:		
½ cup spaghetti		100
*¼ cup marinara sauce		25
1 cup sautéed broccoli	1 cup zucchini	80

* Recipe in Chapter 9

* Recipe in Chapter 9

2 teaspoons butter. . . . . 2 teaspoons olive oil 70

1 cup strawberries. . . . . ¼ melon slice 60

Toni's Treats!

1 slice angel food cake 75

2 tablespoons cool whip 22

1 cup skim or 1 percent fat milk. 95

APPROXIMATE CALORIES: 1,300 FOR THE DAY

 ## NBA Finals Game—Day Two

Basket Breakfast

JUMPBALL	SUBSTITUTIONS	CALORIE COUNT
8 ounces of orange juice	Apple or grapefruit juice.	100
1 toasted English muffin.	Bran or whole-grain muffin	125
2 tablespoons . . . . low-fat cream cheese	2 teaspoons butter.	70
1 cup skim/ . . . . 1 percent fat milk	8 ounces low-fat yogurt.	95/200

Fast-break Lunch

JUMPBALL	SUBSTITUTIONS	CALORIE COUNT
Cheeseburger:		
2–3 ounces lean . . . . ground beef	2–3 ounces ground turkey	200
1 hamburger bun.	2 slices of whole-grain bread.	125
1–2 slices low-fat	Low-fat American or cheddar.	50–80

Swiss cheese

2–3 slices tomato 20

2 tablespoons ketchup . . . . . 2 tablespoons mustard 20

1 cup baby carrots . . . . 1 cup celery sticks. 25

NOTHIN'-BUT-NET DINNER

JUMPBALL	SUBSTITUTIONS	CALORIE COUNT
Beef and vegetable . . . . Chicken stew. . . . . .200/175 stew (1 cup)		
½ cup cooked rice . . . . Couscous. 100		
1 cup salad–mixed greens. 10		
2 tablespoons low-fat dressing 40		
½ cup canned pineapple. . . . . 1 large peach. . . . . .60 (in juice, not syrup)		

TONI'S TREATS!

1 cup pretzels . . . . 2 graham cracker squares 150

1½ ounces low-fat cheese . . . . 8 ounces low-fat yogurt. 115/200

APPROXIMATE CALORIES: 1,600 FOR THE DAY

NBA Finals Game—Day Three

BASKET BREAKFAST

JUMPBALL	SUBSTITUTIONS	CALORIE COUNT
1 cup skim or 1 percent fat milk. 95		
1 or 2 eggs scrambled . . . . Boiled or sunny-side-up 100–200		

2 slices whole-wheat toast. . . . Multigrain or rye. 125

2 teaspoons butter/ . . . . 2 tablespoons low-fat 70
margarine   cream cheese

1 small apple. . . . . 1 small orange. 50

FAST-BREAK LUNCH

JUMPBALL	SUBSTITUTIONS	CALORIE COUNT

Turkey sandwich:

    2–3 ounces turkey . . . . Low-fat bologna. 75/200

    2 slices rye bread. . . . . Whole-grain bread. 125

    2 tablespoons mustard. . . . . 2 teaspoons mayonnaise. 25

    3 slices tomato 15

1 cup carrot or celery sticks . . 1 cup cucumber slices. 25

NOTHIN'-BUT-NET DINNER

JUMPBALL	SUBSTITUTIONS	CALORIE COUNT

*Stir-fry shrimp. . . . . Chicken/lean beef 400

    1 cup shrimp and veggies

½ cup rice (brown is best but white is fine). 100

1 cup cut-up melon. . . . . 1 small orange. 60

TONI'S TREATS!

1 cup corn flakes. . . . . Cheerios 100

1 cup skim or 1 percent fat milk. 95

APPROXIMATE CALORIES: 1,500 FOR THE DAY

* Recipe in Chapter 9

NBA Finals Game—Day Four

BASKET BREAKFAST

JUMPBALL	SUBSTITUTIONS	CALORIE COUNT
1 cup cut-up fruit	1 medium orange	60
½ toasted bagel	2 slices of whole-wheat toast	125
2 tablespoons low-fat cream cheese	2 teaspoons butter or margarine	70

FAST-BREAK LUNCH

JUMPBALL	SUBSTITUTIONS	CALORIE COUNT
Grilled cheese sandwich:		
2 slices multigrain bread		125
2 teaspoons butter or margarine (for grilling)		70
2–3 ounces low-fat cheese		125
1 cup tomato slices		30

NOTHIN'-BUT-NET DINNER

JUMPBALL	SUBSTITUTIONS	CALORIE COUNT
Baked chicken (2–3 ounces) with		110
2 tablespoons barbecue sauce		24
and		
*½ cup macaroni/cheese	1 medium baked potato	165/145
1 cup string beans with	Broccoli, spinach	80
2 teaspoons olive oil		70
8 ounces of fruit juice	1 small-size fresh fruit	100/60

* Recipe in Chapter 9

TONI'S TREATS!

2 graham cracker squares . . . . 2 oatmeal raisin cookies 60/130

1 cup skim or 1 percent fat milk. 85–100

APPROXIMATE CALORIES: 1,300 FOR THE DAY

 # NBA Finals Game—Day Five

BASKET BREAKFAST

JUMPBALL	SUBSTITUTIONS	CALORIE COUNT
2 multigrain waffles 195		
1 cup strawberries.	1 cup blueberries 60	
2–3 tablespoons syrup.	1 tablespoon powdered sugar 140/30	
1 cup skim or 1 percent fat milk. 95		

FAST-BREAK LUNCH

JUMPBALL	SUBSTITUTIONS	CALORIE COUNT
Bologna (2 ounces)	Low-fat cheese/turkey 130/100/50	
(low-fat, cut into squares)		
10 whole-grain crackers.	2 slices whole-grain bread. 125	
2 teaspoons low-fat	2 tablespoons mustard or ketchup . . .25	
mayonnaise		
1 cup tomato slices 30		

NOTHIN'-BUT-NET DINNER

JUMPBALL	SUBSTITUTIONS	CALORIE COUNT
Tacos:		
1–2 taco shells		60–120/
1–2 tortillas		70–140
2–3 ounces ground beef	Ground turkey	200
1–2 ounces low-fat cheese		50–80
½ cup shredded lettuce		5
½ cup cubed tomato		15

TONI'S TREATS!

Banana split:		
1 medium banana		100
1 cup low-fat ice cream	1 cup frozen yogurt	200
1 tablespoon chocolate syrup		40

APPROXIMATE CALORIES: 1,400 FOR THE DAY

 # NBA Finals Game—Day Six

BASKET BREAKFAST

JUMPBALL	SUBSTITUTIONS	CALORIE COUNT
*2 wheat germ pancakes	2 whole-grain waffles	195
1 cup skim or 1 percent fat milk		95
2 teaspoons butter or margarine		70
¼ cup syrup	1 tablespoon powdered sugar	210/50

* Recipe in Chapter 9

FAST-BREAK LUNCH

JUMPBALL	SUBSTITUTIONS	CALORIE COUNT
Hot dog (low-fat):		.130
1 hot dog bun		.125
2 tablespoons mustard	2 tablespoons ketchup	.25
¼ cup sauerkraut (optional)		.7
1 cup baby carrots		.40
1 cup cut-up melon	8 ounces 100-percent fruit juice	.60

NOTHIN'-BUT-NET DINNER

JUMPBALL	SUBSTITUTIONS	CALORIE COUNT
*2–3 oven-fried chicken fingers		.185
* ½ cup oven-fried sweet potato	1 medium baked potato	.175/145
1 cup cooked broccoli (steamed)		.80
(sautéed in 1 teaspoon butter or olive oil)		.35
and		
1 large nectarine	Orange or peach	.60

TONI'S TREATS!

Ice cream sundae:

1 cup low-fat ice cream	1 cup frozen yogurt	.200
¼ cup nuts		.200

APPROXIMATE CALORIES: 1,800 FOR THE DAY

NBA Finals Game—Day Seven

BASKET BREAKFAST

JUMPBALL	SUBSTITUTIONS	CALORIE COUNT
1 medium pear	Any seasonal fruit	.60
½ toasted bagel	1 English muffin	.130
2 tablespoons low-fat cream cheese		.70
1 cup skim or 1 percent fat milk		.95

FAST-BREAK LUNCH

JUMPBALL	SUBSTITUTIONS	CALORIE COUNT
Chicken burrito	Beef burrito	500

NOTHIN'-BUT-NET DINNER

JUMPBALL	SUBSTITUTIONS	CALORIE COUNT
*2–3 ounces slice of turkey meatloaf		.145–220
½ cup mashed potatoes	1 medium baked potato	.125/145
2 tablespoons turkey gravy . . .	2 teaspoons butter or margarine	.15/70
1 cup cooked spinach	1 cup cooked broccoli	.80

TONI'S TREATS!

1 cup Cheerios	Corn flakes	.100
1 cup skim or 1 percent fat milk		.95
½ cup raisins	1 cup fresh berries	.250/60

APPROXIMATE CALORIES: 1,600 FOR THE DAY

* Recipe in Chapter 9

Lacrosse Championship Meal Plans for Kids
Game Day One

CUTTER BREAKFAST

AT THE FACE-OFF	SUBSTITUTIONS	CALORIE COUNT
8 ounces 100-percent fruit juice	Small apple, orange.	100/60
Egg sandwich:		
1 toasted English muffin		130
1–2 scrambled eggs		100–200
1 slice low-fat cheese		40

SLASHING LUNCH

AT THE FACE-OFF	SUBSTITUTIONS	CALORIE COUNT
Tuna salad sandwich:		
2–3 ounces tuna (in water)	3 ounces chicken	110
2 slices of multigrain bread	Whole-wheat or rye bread.	125
1 cup baby carrots	1 cup cucumber slices.	25

SHOOTING DINNER

AT THE FACE-OFF	SUBSTITUTIONS	CALORIE COUNT
*Turkey meatloaf (2–3 ounces).		145–220
½ cup mashed potatoes	1 medium baked potato	160/145
1 cup string beans	Broccoli, zucchini	40
2 teaspoons olive oil	Butter or margarine	70
and		
1 cup skim or 1 percent fat milk.		95

* Recipe in Chapter 9

TONI'S TREATS!

1 cup low-fat . . . . 1 cup frozen yogurt 200
vanilla yogurt

1 cup fresh berries 60

APPROXIMATE CALORIES: 1,500 FOR THE DAY

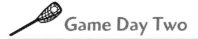 Game Day Two

CUTTER BREAKFAST

AT THE FACE-OFF	SUBSTITUTIONS	CALORIE COUNT
8 ounces 100-percent fruit juice	Any small fruit	100/60
1 cup Cheerios	1 cup corn flakes	100
1 cup skim or 1 percent fat milk		95

SLASHING LUNCH

AT THE FACE-OFF	SUBSTITUTIONS	CALORIE COUNT
Roast beef sandwich:		
2–3 ounces roast beef	2–3 ounces turkey	160/75
1 whole-grain roll	2 slices rye bread	125
2 teaspoons low-fat mayonnaise	2 tablespoons mustard	25
1 cup tomato slices		15
½ cup lettuce		5
1 cup cut-up fruit		60

SHOOTING DINNER

AT THE FACE-OFF	SUBSTITUTIONS	CALORIE COUNT
Baked chicken (2–3 ounces) . . 3 ounces baked fish. 110		
2 tablespoons barbecue sauce. 24		
1 cup cooked broccoli . . . . Spinach, cauliflower 40		
1 teaspoon olive oil. 35		
1 cup cooked rice (brown is best but white is fine) 200		

TONI'S TREATS!

Fruit sundae:

> 1 cup low-fat ice cream . . . . 1 cup low-fat frozen yogurt. 200
>
> ½ cup cut-up fresh fruit. 50
>
> 1 tablespoon chocolate syrup 40

APPROXIMATE CALORIES: 1,300 FOR THE DAY

Game Day Three

CUTTER BREAKFAST

AT THE FACE-OFF	SUBSTITUTIONS	CALORIE COUNT
2 whole-grain waffles 195		
2–3 tablespoons syrup. . . . . . . 1 tablespoon powered sugar 140/30		
1 cup strawberries. . . . . 1 cup blueberries 60		
1 cup skim or 1 percent fat milk. 95		

SLASHING LUNCH

AT THE FACE-OFF	SUBSTITUTIONS	CALORIE COUNT
1 cup tomato soup..........	1 cup chicken or vegetable soup.....85	

and

Egg salad sandwich:

| 2 slices multigrain bread . . . | Whole-wheat or rye bread..........125 | |
| ½ cup egg salad..350 | | |

SHOOTING DINNER

AT THE FACE-OFF	SUBSTITUTIONS	CALORIE COUNT
*Not-so-sloppy turkey Joes:		
2–3 ounces of turkey Joes....................................185		
1 whole-grain roll..125		
2 cups tossed salad.........	1 cup tomato and cucumber slices . . .25	
2 tablespoons low-fat dressing 40		
1 cup baked potato chips....................................50		

TONI'S TREATS!

Banana split:

1 banana 100		
1 cup low-fat ice cream	1 cup low-fat yogurt 200	
1 tablespoon chocolate syrup 40		

APPROXIMATE CALORIES: 1,700 FOR THE DAY

* Recipe in Chapter 9

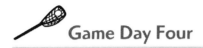

Game Day Four

CUTTER BREAKFAST

AT THE FACE-OFF	SUBSTITUTIONS	CALORIE COUNT
1 cup corn flakes	1 cup Cheerios	110
1 cup fresh berries	1 small banana	60
1 cup low-fat milk		95

SLASHING LUNCH

AT THE FACE-OFF	SUBSTITUTIONS	CALORIE COUNT
Hot dog:		
1 Hot dog	1 low-fat hot dog	190/130
1 hot dog bun		125
2 tablespoons mustard	2 tablespoons ketchup	25
½ cup sauerkraut (optional)		15
1 cup baby carrots		20

SHOOTING DINNER

AT THE FACE-OFF	SUBSTITUTIONS	CALORIE COUNT
*Chicken stir-fry:		
1 cup stir-fried chicken and veggies	Shrimp, lean beef	400
1 cup cooked rice (brown is best but white is fine)		200
1 orange	1 cup fresh pineapple	60

* Recipe in Chapter 9

TONI'S TREATS!

1 cup skim or . . . . 1 cup low-fat yogurt 95/200
1 percent fat milk

2 graham cracker squares. 60

APPROXIMATE CALORIES: 1,400 FOR THE DAY

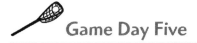 Game Day Five

CUTTER BREAKFAST

AT THE FACE-OFF	SUBSTITUTIONS	CALORIE COUNT
1 cup berries 60		
*2 wheat germ pancakes. . . . . 2 whole-grain waffles 195		
3 tablespoons syrup . . . . 1 tablespoons powdered sugar 140/30		
1 egg any style. 100		

SLASHING LUNCH

AT THE FACE-OFF	SUBSTITUTIONS	CALORIE COUNT
Thin-crust pizza with veggie topping (1 slice) 195		
1 cup Jell-O with cut-up fruit 160		
1 cup skim or 1 percent fat milk. 95		

* Recipe in Chapter 9

SHOOTING DINNER

AT THE FACE-OFF	SUBSTITUTIONS	CALORIE COUNT
Cheeseburger:		
2–3 ounce lean ground beef	2–3 ounces ground turkey	150–200
1–2 slices low-fat cheese		50–80
1 hamburger bun	2 slices whole-wheat bread	125
2 teaspoons low-fat mayonnaise	2 tablespoons ketchup	30
2 slices tomato		10
1 cup baby carrots		40

TONI'S TREATS!

1 slice whole-grain bread	5 crackers	125
2 tablespoons peanut butter		190
¼ cup raisins		110

APPROXIMATE CALORIES: 1,800 FOR THE DAY

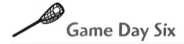 Game Day Six

CUTTER BREAKFAST

AT THE FACE-OFF	SUBSTITUTIONS	CALORIE COUNT
1 cup cut-up melon		60
1 cup low-fat yogurt	1 cup skim or 1 percent fat milk	200/95
½ toasted bagel	2 slices whole-wheat toast	125
1–2 slices low-fat cheese		50–80

SLASHING LUNCH

AT THE FACE-OFF	SUBSTITUTIONS	CALORIE COUNT

Dunking chicken:

2–3 ounces grilled chicken strips 115

2 tablespoons barbecue sauce for dunking 24

1 medium baked potato. 145

2 tablespoons low-fat . . . . 2 teaspoons butter or margarine. 50/70
sour cream

SHOOTING DINNER

AT THE FACE-OFF	SUBSTITUTIONS	CALORIE COUNT

*Beef and vegetable . . . . Chicken stew. 200/175
stew (1 cup)

1 cup cooked rice (brown is best but white is fine) 200

2 cups salad–mixed greens 25

2 tablespoons low-fat dressing 40

½ cup chocolate pudding (reduced fat) 100

TONI'S TREATS!

1 cup Cheerios . . . . Corn flakes .100

1 cup skim or . . . . 1 cup low-fat yogurt 95/200
1 percent fat milk

1 small banana, sliced. 90

APPROXIMATE CALORIES: 1,700 FOR THE DAY

* Recipe in Chapter 9

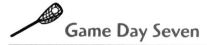 **Game Day Seven**

CUTTER BREAKFAST

AT THE FACE-OFF	SUBSTITUTIONS	CALORIE COUNT
1 cup cut-up strawberries	½ cup blueberries	.60
1 cup low-fat yogurt	1 cup skim or 1 percent fat milk. . . .	.200/95
2 slices rye toast	Multigrain or whole-wheat	.125
2 tablespoons low-fat cream cheese or		
2 teaspoons butter or margarine.		.70

SLASHING LUNCH

AT THE FACE-OFF	SUBSTITUTIONS	CALORIE COUNT
Tuna melt:		
3 ounces tuna (canned in water).		.110
2 tablespoons low-fat mayonnaise.		.75
1 English muffin, toasted.		.125
2 slices low-fat cheese		.75
1 cup cucumber slices.	1 cup celery sticks.	.15

SHOOTING DINNER

AT THE FACE-OFF	SUBSTITUTIONS	CALORIE COUNT
*Spaghetti and meat sauce:		
1 cup spaghetti.	Any other type pasta.	.200
1 cup meat sauce.		.140
2 cups mixed green salad	1 cup cooked broccoli	.25
2 tablespoons low-fat salad dressing.		.40

* Recipe in Chapter 9

Toni's Treats!

Banana split:

   1 cup low-fat ice cream . . . . 1 cup low-fat frozen yogurt 200

   1 sliced banana (small) 90

   1 tablespoons chocolate syrup. 40

APPROXIMATE CALORIES: 1,500 FOR THE DAY

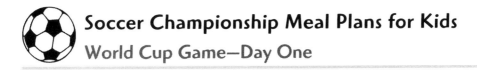

Soccer Championship Meal Plans for Kids
World Cup Game—Day One

Header Breakfast

AT THE FACE-OFF	SUBSTITUTIONS	CALORIE COUNT
1 cup fruit/yogurt smoothie:		
Blend:		
1 cup low-fat vanilla yogurt. 200		
1 cup berries, banana or other fruit 60		
1 English muffin, toasted . . . . Bran or whole-grain 125		
2 teaspoons butter/margarine or		
2 tablespoons low-fat cream cheese 70		

Sweeper Lunch

AT THE FACE-OFF	SUBSTITUTIONS	CALORIE COUNT
Grilled chicken sandwich:		
2 slices bread, Multigrain, whole-wheat, or rye 125		
2–3 ounces grilled chicken . . . 2–3 ounces turkey. 140/75		

2 teaspoons butter/margarine or
2 tablespoons low-fat cream cheese 70

2 teaspoons low-fat . . . . 2 tablespoons mustard 25
mayonnaise

1 cup sliced tomato . . . . 1 cup baby carrots. 25

8 ounces 100-percent. . . . . . . 8 ounces vegetable juice 100/45
fruit juice

BREAKAWAY DINNER

AT THE FACE-OFF	SUBSTITUTIONS	CALORIE COUNT
*Beef and vegetable . . . . 1 cup chicken stew . . . . .200/175 stew (1 cup)		
½ cup cooked rice (brown is best but white is fine). 100		
2 cups salad—mixed greens 25		
2 tablespoons low-fat dressing 40		

TONI'S TREATS!

1 cup low-fat yogurt . . . . 1 cup low-fat ice cream. 200

1 medium banana, sliced . . . . ¼ cup raisins. 100

APPROXIMATE CALORIES: 1,400 FOR THE DAY

⚽ World Cup Game—Day Two

HEADER BREAKFAST

AT THE FACE-OFF	SUBSTITUTIONS	CALORIE COUNT
¾ cup raisin bran . . . . 1 cup Cheerios, Rice Krispies 100		

* Recipe in Chapter 9

1 slice rye bread, toasted. . . . . Whole-wheat, multigrain 60

1 egg, scrambled . . . . Poached, fried 100

2 teaspoons butter/margarine or
2 tablespoons low-fat cream cheese 70

1 cup skim or 1 percent fat milk. 95

SWEEPER LUNCH

AT THE FACE-OFF	SUBSTITUTIONS	CALORIE COUNT
Thin-crust pizza with veggie topping (1 slice) 195		
1 cup cut-up fruit . . . . 1 small apple, peach 60		
1 cup skim or 1 percent fat milk. 95		

BREAKAWAY DINNER

AT THE FACE-OFF	SUBSTITUTIONS	CALORIE COUNT
*Turkey meatloaf (2–3 ounces). 145–220		
1 medium baked potato. . . . . . ½ cup mashed potato 145/160		
1 cup cooked broccoli . . . . String beans, zucchini. 80		
1 teaspoon butter or oil. 35		

TONI'S TREATS!

2 graham cracker squares . . . . 5 whole-grain crackers 65

1 cup skim or 1 percent fat milk. 95

1 cup grapes 60

APPROXIMATE CALORIES: 1,400 FOR THE DAY

* Recipe in Chapter 9

⚽ World Cup Game—Day Three

HEADER BREAKFAST

AT THE FACE-OFF	SUBSTITUTIONS	CALORIE COUNT
½ cup cooked cereal	Oatmeal, farina, Cream-of-Wheat	70
¼ cup raisins	¼ cup dried cranberries	110
1 cup skim or 1 percent fat milk		95
1 teaspoon butter or margarine		35

SWEEPER LUNCH

AT THE FACE-OFF	SUBSTITUTIONS	CALORIE COUNT
Bologna and cheese sandwich:		
2 slices low-fat American cheese		40
2 slices low-fat bologna		130
2 slices multigrain bread	Whole-wheat or rye	125
2 teaspoons low-fat mayonnaise or 2 tablespoons mustard		25
1 cup chicken soup		80
1 cup cucumber slices	1 cup celery sticks, baby carrots	15

BREAKAWAY DINNER

AT THE FACE-OFF	SUBSTITUTIONS	CALORIE COUNT
*Spaghetti and meat sauce:		
1 cup cooked spaghetti		200
1 cup meat sauce		140
2 cups mixed greens		25
2 tablespoons low-fat dressing		50

* Recipe in Chapter 9

Toni's Treats!

Thin-crust cheese pizza (1 slice). 195

1 cup fresh fruit. . . . . Banana slices, cut-up peaches 60

APPROXIMATE CALORIES: 1,400 FOR THE DAY

 # World Cup Game—Day Four

Header Breakfast

AT THE FACE-OFF	SUBSTITUTIONS	CALORIE COUNT
1 waffle, whole-grain preferred.		.100
1 cup berries	1 cup other fresh fruit.	.60
3 tablespoons syrup	1 tablespoons powdered sugar	.140/30
1 cup skim or 1 percent fat milk.		.95

Sweeper Lunch

AT THE FACE-OFF	SUBSTITUTIONS	CALORIE COUNT
Turkey and Swiss sandwich:		
2 slices turkey	Roast beef	.50/130
2 slices Swiss cheese		.100
2 slices rye bread.	Multigrain, whole-wheat.	.125
2 tablespoons mustard.		.20
1/4 melon wedge	1 small orange.	.60

BREAKAWAY DINNER

AT THE FACE-OFF	SUBSTITUTIONS	CALORIE COUNT
Baked chicken (2–3 ounces)		100

(marinate in Italian dressing for about 20 minutes before baking)

and

1½ cups cooked string bean	Broccoli	120
*Macaroni and cheese (½ cup)		165

TONI'S TREATS!

1 cup frozen yogurt	1 cup low-fat ice cream	200
2 graham cracker squares		65
crumbled and poured over yogurt or ice cream		
2 tablespoons chocolate syrup		40

APPROXIMATE CALORIES: 1,500 FOR THE DAY

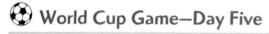 ## World Cup Game—Day Five

HEADER BREAKFAST

AT THE FACE-OFF	SUBSTITUTIONS	CALORIE COUNT
½ toasted bagel	1 English muffin	125
2 tablespoons peanut butter		190
2 tablespoons low-sugar jelly		50
1 cup berries	1 cup other fresh fruit	60
1 cup skim or 1 percent fat milk		95

* Recipe in Chapter 9

SWEEPER LUNCH

AT THE FACE-OFF	SUBSTITUTIONS	CALORIE COUNT

Cheeseburger:

1 hamburger roll	2 slices whole-wheat bread 125	
2–3 ounce lean	Ground turkey. 200	
ground beef		
2–3 slices of tomato 20		
2 teaspoons low-fat	1 tablespoon mustard or ketchup . . .25	
mayonnaise		

1 cup baby carrots, celery sticks, or cucumber slices. 25

BREAKAWAY DINNER

AT THE FACE-OFF	SUBSTITUTIONS	CALORIE COUNT

*Veggie baked ziti (1½ cups) 380		
2 cups mixed greens 25		
2 tablespoons low-fat 40		
salad dressing		
1 small apple	1 small banana 60/90	

TONI'S TREATS!

| 2 ounces low-fat cheese . . . . .125 | | |
| 5 whole-grain crackers . . . . . . | 1 slice whole-grain bread . . . . .125 | |

APPROXIMATE CALORIES: 1,700 FOR THE DAY

* Recipe in Chapter 9

⚽ World Cup Game—Day Six

HEADER BREAKFAST

AT THE FACE-OFF	SUBSTITUTIONS	CALORIE COUNT
1 cup corn flakes	Cheerios, Rice Krispies	100
1 small banana	¼ cup raisins	90/110
1 cup skim or 1 percent fat milk		95

SWEEPER LUNCH

AT THE FACE-OFF	SUBSTITUTIONS	CALORIE COUNT
Hot dog:		
Hot dog (low-fat):		130
1 hot dog bun		125
½ cup sauerkraut (optional)		15
2 tablespoons mustard	2 tablespoons ketchup	25
1 cup baby carrots		40
2 tablespoons low-fat dressing		40

BREAKAWAY DINNER

AT THE FACE-OFF	SUBSTITUTIONS	CALORIE COUNT
*Stir-fried chicken:		
1 cup chicken and veggie stir-fry	Shrimp or lean beef and veggie	400
1 cup rice (brown rice is best but white is fine)		200

* Recipe in Chapter 9

Toni's Treats!

1 cup low-fat yogurt . . . . 1 cup low-fat ice cream. 200

1 cup cut-up fruit 60

APPROXIMATE CALORIES: 1,500 FOR THE DAY

World Cup Game—Day Seven

Header Breakfast

AT THE FACE-OFF	SUBSTITUTIONS	CALORIE COUNT
1–2 scrambled eggs	Sunny-side-up or boiled	100/200
1–2 slices of toast	Multigrain, whole-wheat or rye	60–125
½ cup home fries	½ cup French fries	125
2 strips bacon		60
8 ounces 100-percent fruit juice	Fresh fruit	100

Sweeper Lunch

AT THE FACE-OFF	SUBSTITUTIONS	CALORIE COUNT
Turkey sandwich:		
2 ounces turkey	Turkey bologna	50/130
2 slices rye bread	Whole-grain	125
2 tablespoons mustard	2 teaspoons low-fat mayo	25
3 slices tomato		
1 cup baby carrots	1 cup cucumber slices	25
1 cup skim or 1 percent fat milk		95

BREAKAWAY DINNER

AT THE FACE-OFF	SUBSTITUTIONS	CALORIE COUNT
*Oven-fried chicken fingers (2–3 ounces)		185
*1 cup oven-fried sweet potato	1 medium baked potato	350/145
1 cup cooked broccoli	Spinach, zucchini	80
1 teaspoon butter or olive oil		35
1 small orange	1 cup canned fruit (in its own juice, not syrup)	60/100

TONI'S TREATS!

1 cup skim or 1 percent fat milk		95
2 graham cracker squares		65

APPROXIMATE CALORIES: 1,700 FOR THE DAY

* Recipe in Chapter 9

All-Star Meal Plans for Super-Active Kids

(For example: tennis, ballet, swim, track, hockey, gymnastics, volleyball, and field hockey.)

All Star—Day One

SET-POINT BREAKFAST

ON THE GO	SUBSTITUTIONS	CALORIE COUNT
1 small banana	8 ounces orange juice	100
1 cup Cheerios	Any non-frosted cereal	100
8 ounces low-fat milk	8 ounces low-fat yogurt	95/200

PLIÉ LUNCH

ON THE GO	SUBSTITUTIONS	CALORIE COUNT
Tuna salad sandwich:		
2–3 ounces tuna (canned in water)	2–3 ounces chicken	110
2 tablespoons low-fat mayonnaise		75
1 medium tomato, sliced		25
½ cup shredded lettuce		5
1 whole-grain roll	2 slices rye bread	125

DOLPHIN-KICK DINNER

ON THE GO	SUBSTITUTIONS	CALORIE COUNT
Baked chicken (3 ounces) (marinated in Italian dressing 20 minutes before baking)		110
Spaghetti marinara:		
1 cup spaghetti		200
*½ cup marinara sauce		50

* Recipe in Chapter 9

1 cup sautéed broccoli. . . . . . . 1 cup zucchini, string beans 80

2 teaspoons butter. . . . . 2 teaspoons olive oil 70

1 cup strawberries. . . . . ¼ melon slice 60

TONI'S TREATS!

1 slice angel food cake 75

2 tablespoons Cool Whip. 20

1 cup skim or 1 percent fat milk. 95

APPROXIMATE CALORIES: 1,400 FOR THE DAY

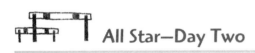 All Star—Day Two

HURDLE BREAKFAST

ON THE GO	SUBSTITUTIONS	CALORIE COUNT
1–2 scrambled eggs	Sunny-side-up or boiled	100–200
1–2 slices of toast	Multigrain, whole-wheat, or rye	.60–125
½ cup home fries	½ cup French fries	125
2 strips bacon		.50
8 ounces 100-percent fruit juice	Orange, apple, etc.	100

HAT-TRICK LUNCH

ON THE GO	SUBSTITUTIONS	CALORIE COUNT
Turkey sandwich:		
2 ounces turkey	Turkey bologna	.50/130
2 slices rye bread	Whole-grain.	.125

2 tablespoons mustard . . . . . 2 teaspoons low-fat mayo 25

3 slices tomato

1 cup baby carrots . . . . 1 cup cucumber slices 25

1 cup skim or 1 percent fat milk 95

ROUND-OFF DINNER

ON THE GO	SUBSTITUTIONS	CALORIE COUNT
*2–3 ounces oven-fried chicken fingers	. . . .	.185
*1 cup oven-fried sweet potato	. . . . 1 medium baked potato	. . . . .350/145
1 cup cooked broccoli	. . . . Spinach, zucchini	80
1 teaspoon butter or olive oil	. . . .	.35
1 small orange	. . . . 1 cup canned fruit (in its own juice not syrup)	. . . . 60/100

TONI'S TREATS!

1 cup skim or 1 percent fat milk 95

2 graham cracker squares 65

APPROXIMATE CALORIES: 1,700 FOR THE DAY

* Recipe in Chapter 9

All Star—Day Three

SPIKE BREAKFAST

ON THE GO	SUBSTITUTIONS	CALORIE COUNT

1 cup fruit/yogurt smoothie:

Blend:

    1 cup low-fat vanilla yogurt 200

    1 cup berries, banana or other fruit. 60

1 English muffin, toasted . . . . Bran or whole-grain 125

2 teaspoons butter/ margarine or
2 tablespoons low-fat cream cheese 70

FLICK LUNCH

ON THE GO	SUBSTITUTIONS	CALORIE COUNT

1 cup tomato soup. . . . . 1 cup chicken or vegetable soup. 80

Grilled cheese sandwich:

    2 slices multigrain bread . . . Whole-wheat or rye bread. 125

    ½ cup egg salad 350

    1 cup tomato slices 30

2 teaspoons butter or margarine for grilling. 70

SINGLES DINNER

ON THE GO	SUBSTITUTIONS	CALORIE COUNT

*Not-so-sloppy turkey Joes:

    2–3 ounces of turkey Joes 185

    1 whole-grain roll. 125

2 cups tossed salad . . . . 1 cup tomato and cucumber slices . . .25

2 tablespoons low-fat dressing 40

* Recipe in Chapter 9

Toni's Treats!

Banana split:

1 medium banana 100

1 cup low-fat ice cream . . . . 1 cup low-fat yogurt 200

1 tablespoons chocolate syrup. 40

APPROXIMATE CALORIES: 1,800 FOR THE DAY

 ## All Star—Day Four

Parallel-bar Breakfast

ON THE GO	SUBSTITUTIONS	CALORIE COUNT
1 cup berries 60		
*2 Wheat germ pancakes . . . . 2 whole-grain waffles 195		
3 tablespoons syrup . . . . 1 tablespoons powdered sugar 140/30		
1 egg any style. 100		

Sprint Lunch

ON THE GO	SUBSTITUTIONS	CALORIE COUNT
Thin-crust pizza with veggie topping (1 slice) 195		
1 cup Jell-O with cut-up fruit 160		
1 cup skim or 1 percent fat milk. 95		

Slap Shot Dinner

ON THE GO	SUBSTITUTIONS	CALORIE COUNT
Cheeseburger:		
2–3 ounce lean 2–3 ounces ground turkey .200		
ground beef		

1–2 slices low-fat cheese 50–80

1 hamburger bun . . . . 2 slices whole-wheat bread 125

2 teaspoons low-fat . . . . 2 tablespoons ketchup. 25
mayonnaise

2 slices tomato 10

1 cup baby carrots 40

Toni's Treats!

1 slice whole-grain bread . . . . 5 crackers 125

2 tablespoons peanut butter 190

¼ cup raisins. 110

APPROXIMATE CALORIES: 1,700 FOR THE DAY

All Star—Day Five

Knee-pad Breakfast

ON THE GO	SUBSTITUTIONS	CALORIE COUNT
1 cup cut-up melon 60		
1 cup low-fat yogurt . . . . 1 cup skim or 1 percent fat milk. 200/95		
½ toasted bagel . . . . 2 slices whole-wheat toast. 125		
1–2 slices low-fat cheese 50–80		

Scoop Lunch

ON THE GO	SUBSTITUTIONS	CALORIE COUNT
Dunking chicken:		
2–3 ounces of grilled chicken strips 115		
2 tablespoons barbecue sauce for dunking .24		

1 medium baked potato. 145

2 tablespoons low-fat sour cream or
2 teaspoons butter or margarine. 50/70

BUTTERFLY DINNER

ON THE GO	SUBSTITUTIONS	CALORIE COUNT
*1 cup beef and . . . . Chicken stew. . . . . .200/175 vegetable stew		
1 cup cooked rice (brown is best but white is fine) 200		
2 cup salad—mixed greens 25		
2 tablespoons low-fat dressing 40		
1/2 cup chocolate pudding (reduced fat) 100		

TONI'S TREATS!

1 cup Cheerios . . . . Corn flakes .100		
1 cup skim . . . . 1 cup low-fat yogurt . . . . .95/200 or 1 percent fat milk		
1 small banana 90		

APPROXIMATE CALORIES: 1,600 FOR THE DAY

* Recipe in Chapter 9

All Star—Day Six

MARATHON BREAKFAST

ON THE GO	SUBSTITUTIONS	CALORIE COUNT
1 cup cut-up strawberries . . . . 1 cup blueberries 60		
1 cup low-fat yogurt . . . . 1 cup skim or 1 percent fat milk. 200/95		
2 slices rye toast . . . . Multigrain or whole-wheat 125		
2 tablespoons low-fat cream cheese or 2 teaspoons butter/margarine 70		

HAND-SPRING LUNCH

ON THE GO	SUBSTITUTIONS	CALORIE COUNT
Tuna melt:		
3 ounces tuna (canned in water). 110		
2 tablespoons low-fat mayonnaise. 75		
1 English muffin, toasted. 125		
2 slices low-fat cheese 75		
1 cup cucumber slices. . . . . . . 1 cup celery sticks. 15		

RELAY-RACE DINNER

ON THE GO	SUBSTITUTIONS	CALORIE COUNT
*Stir-fried chicken:		
1 cup chicken Shrimp or lean beef and veggie . . . . .400 and veggie stir-fry		
1 cup rice (brown rice is best but white is fine) 200		

* Recipe in Chapter 9

TONI'S TREATS!

Banana split:

1 cup low-fat ice cream . . . . 1 cup low-fat frozen yogurt 200

1 sliced banana 110

1 tablespoon chocolate syrup 40

APPROXIMATE CALORIES: 1,700 FOR THE DAY

 ## All Star—Day Seven

RELEVÉ BREAKFAST

ON THE GO	SUBSTITUTIONS	CALORIE COUNT
½ toasted bagel . . . . 1 English muffin 125		
2 tablespoons peanut butter 190		
2 tablespoons low-sugar preserves 50		
1 cup berries . . . . 1 cup other fresh fruit. 60		
1 cup skim or 1 percent fat milk. 95		

GOALIE LUNCH

ON THE GO	SUBSTITUTIONS	CALORIE COUNT

Cheeseburger:

1 hamburger roll . . . . 2 slices whole-wheat bread 125

2–3 ounce lean . . . . Ground turkey. 200
ground beef

2–3 slices of tomato 20

1–2 slices of low-fat cheese 50–80

2 teaspoons low-fat . . . . 2 tablespoons mustard or ketchup . . .25
mayonnaise

1 cup baby carrots . . . . 1 cup celery sticks/ 25
cucumber slices

Net Dinner

ON THE GO	SUBSTITUTIONS	CALORIE COUNT

*Veggie baked ziti (1 ½ cups) 380

2 cups mixed greens 25

2 tablespoons low-fat salad dressing 40

1 small apple . . . . 1 small banana 60/90

Toni's Treats!

2 ounces low-fat cheese 125

5 whole-grain crackers . . . . . . 1 slice whole-grain bread 125

APPROXIMATE CALORIES: 1,700 FOR THE DAY

* Recipe in Chapter 9

child-friendly recipes that are good for the whole family*

TONI COLARUSSO, M.S.

Chicken and Vegetable Stir-Fry

This can also be made by substituting shrimp or lean beef for chicken. Use fish or vegetable broth, and beef broth when cooking beef.

3 teaspoons olive oil, divided

Cooking spray

1½ pounds (24 ounces) chicken breast, cut into 1-inch strips

1½ cup sliced shallots

1½ cup green pepper cut in strips

6 garlic cloves, minced

6 cups of your favorite mushrooms, sliced

3 tablespoons low-sodium soy sauce

1½ cup salt-free chicken broth

3 tablespoon chopped fresh basil

Salt and pepper to taste

4½ cups hot cooked rice

Heat ½ teaspoon oil in a nonstick skillet or wok coated with cooking spray. Use medium high heat until hot. Add chicken; stir-fry 2 minutes. Remove chicken and set aside. Wipe skillet clean with a paper towel.

Heat ½ teaspoon oil in the skilled. Add shallots, pepper strips, and garlic; stir-fry for 1 minute. Stir in soy-flavored water; cook 1 minute. Add broth; reduce heat

* PDFs of all recipes can be downloaded from www.drrobsays.com.

and simmer 3 minutes. Add the chicken; cook 1 minute. Stir in basil, salt, and pepper.

Yield: 6 servings

High-Energy Meat Loaf

This unique, two-protein recipe is moist and flavorful. You might consider doubling the ingredients and making two loaves, so you can save one in the freezer for later.

Cooking spray

1 cup finely chopped onion

3 garlic cloves, minced

1 cup bread crumbs

½ cup fat-free milk

1 tablespoon barbecue sauce

1 teaspoon salt

½ teaspoon freshly ground black pepper

4 large egg whites

1½ pounds ground turkey breast

½ pound extra lean ground beef

Two 10-ounce packages of frozen leaf spinach; thawed, drained, and squeezed dry

½ cup ketchup

Preheat oven to 350 degrees.

Coat a large nonstick skillet with cooking spray and heat over medium-high heat. Add onion. Sauté 4 minutes. Add garlic; sauté 30 seconds. Remove from heat. Combine the onion/garlic mixture with the rest of the ingredients; mix well.

Make a loaf shape, and place it on a broiler pan coated with cooking spray. Coat the loaf with ketchup. Bake at 350 degrees for 45 minutes, or until a thermometer registers 160 degrees.

Wait 10 minutes before slicing.

Yield: 8 single slice servings

Macaroni and Cheese for Kids

Let the kids help make this one. Once they taste it, they'll never eat the boxed stuff again.

1 tablespoon butter or margarine

2 tablespoons whole-wheat flour

1¼ cups low-fat milk

1½ cups reduced fat shredded cheddar cheese

3 tablespoons grated Parmesan cheese

1 teaspoon low-sodium Worcestershire sauce

½ teaspoon dry mustard

⅛ teaspoon ground pepper

½ teaspoon salt

4 cups hot cooked elbow macaroni (cook 1¾ cups dry macaroni)

Melt butter/margarine in a saucepan over medium heat; add flour and cook 1 minute, stirring constantly with a wire whisk. Continue stirring as you gradually add milk. Bring to a boil and cook 1 minute as you continue to stir. Remove from heat; add cheeses and all other ingredients except the macaroni. Stir until the cheeses melt. Combine the cheese sauce and macaroni in a bowl. Stir well, and serve immediately.

Yield: 6 servings (¾ cup per person)

Beef and Vegetable Stew

This can also be made by substituting 1 pound of chicken for beef, and using chicken broth instead of beef broth. If you make the stew in a crock-pot, you'll be able to go to the game with the kids because, by the time you return, the stew will be ready to serve.

2 cans (14¼-ounce size) fat-free beef broth

1 pound lean, boned chuck roast

1 teaspoon olive oil, divided

4 cups vertically sliced onion

½ cup crushed tomatoes

3 garlic cloves, minced

3 cups carrots, cubed

3 cups red potatoes, cubed

2 ½ cups mushrooms, quartered

½ cup dry red wine or nonalcoholic red wine

1 teaspoon salt

¼ teaspoon pepper

One 10-ounce package frozen green peas, thawed

2 tablespoons water

1 tablespoon cornstarch

Fresh parsley, chopped (optional garnish

Bring the beef broth to a boil in a small saucepan; cook 15 minutes, or until reduced to 2 cups. Set aside.

Trim fat from beef and cut into ½-inch cubes. Heat ½ teaspoon oil in a large Dutch oven over medium high heat. Add beef; brown on one side. Remove from pan and set aside. Heat remaining oil in pan over medium high heat. Add onion, crushed tomatoes, and garlic; cook 5 minutes, stirring constantly. Return beef to pan. Add reduced broth, and next six ingredients (carrots through peas). Bring to a boil. Cover, and reduce heat. Simmer 45 minutes or until vegetables are tender.

Combine water and cornstarch in a small bowl; stir well. Add to stew. Bring to a boil; cook 1 minute, stirring constantly. Ladle into soup bowls, and garnish with parsley (optional).

Yield: 8 servings (serving size: approximately 1 cup)

Chicken Fingers with Sweet and Sour Dipping Sauce

If your kids think they like restaurant-made chicken nuggets, wait until they taste these!

Sauce:

¼ cup honey

¼ cup Dijon mustard

To prepare sauce, combine the two ingredients in a small bowl, cover, and chill. Alternate: Use ½ cup of your favorite barbecue sauce.

Chicken:

1½ pounds chicken breast tenders (16 pieces)

½ cup skim or 1 percent milk

½ cup coarsely crushed cornflakes

¼ cup seasoned bread crumbs

1 tablespoon instant minced onion

1 teaspoon paprika

¼ teaspoon dried thyme

¼ teaspoon black pepper

½ teaspoon salt

1 tablespoon vegetable oil

Preheat oven to 400 degrees.

Combine chicken and milk in a shallow dish, cover, and chill for 15 minutes. Drain chicken, discarding milk.

Combine cornflakes, bread crumbs, onion, paprika, thyme, and pepper in a large zip-top plastic bag; add 4 pieces of chicken. Seal and shake to coat the chicken. Repeat the procedure until all the chicken is coated.

Spread oil evenly on a jelly roll pan, and arrange chicken in a single layer. Bake at 400 degrees for 4 minutes on each side or until done.

Serve with sauce.

Yield: 8 servings

Sweet Potato Crisps

We all know that French fries aren't good for us. Here's a healthy substitute that kids will like.

4 medium sweet potatoes, peeled and cut into ¼ inch slices

1 tablespoon olive oil

¼ teaspoon salt

¼ teaspoon ground pepper

Vegetable cooking spray

1 tablespoon finely chopped fresh parsley

Combine the potatoes, olive oil, salt, and pepper in a large bowl, and toss gently to coat. Arrange the sweet potato slices in a single layer on a large baking sheet coated with cooking spray. Bake at 400 degrees for 20–25 minutes (turn after 15 minutes) or until tender.

Yield: 7 servings (½ cup per person)

All-American Tomato Sauce

Use your favorite Italian pasta, and try this quick and easy tomato sauce that beats anything out of a can or jar. This is another recipe that can be made in batches to save in the freezer. It can also be part of a meat sauce; just use this recipe, but, as a first step, brown 1½ pounds of extra-lean ground beef or ground turkey; drain it, and then add to tomato sauce with the rest of the ingredients.

1 tablespoon olive oil

1½ cups chopped onion

1 teaspoon dried oregano

4 garlic cloves, minced

½ cup water

1 teaspoon dried basil

½ teaspoon salt

¼ teaspoon fresh ground black pepper

Two 28-ounce cans crushed tomatoes, undrained

One 6-ounce can tomato paste

Heat oil in a large saucepan over medium heat. Add onion and garlic. Cook until tender, about 5–6 minutes. Add crushed tomatoes, tomato paste, oregano, and basil. Cook 10–15 more minutes. Stir occasionally. Season with salt and pepper.

Yield: 8 cups (1 cup per person)

Post-game Pancakes

Wouldn't the family love a pancake party after the game? If you mix a batch of the dry ingredients prior to game time, you can have your game—and eat well later in no more time than it takes to make frozen pancakes. And here's the best news: not only does the wheat germ add a nutty flavor, it also adds more iron, zinc, and folate.

1¼ cups all-purpose flour

¼ cup whole-wheat flour

½ cup toasted or honey-crunch wheat germ

2 teaspoons honey

1 teaspoon baking soda

¼ teaspoon salt

2 cups 1 percent milk

2 large egg whites

Cooking spray

Combine the flours with wheat germ, honey, baking soda, and salt in a large bowl. Combine the milk and egg whites, and add the liquid to the flour mixture, stirring until smooth.

Spoon ¼ cup of batter on a hot nonstick griddle (or a large nonstick skillet) coated with cooking spray. Turn the pancakes when the tops are covered with bubbles and the edges look cooked. Cook for 1–2 minutes more on the other side.

Yield: 12 pancakes

Touchdown Joes

This is our version of sloppy Joes, a favorite when we were kids.

¾ cup chopped onion

½ cup chopped green pepper

¾ pound ground round beef or ground turkey

2 cups canned, crushed tomatoes

2 tablespoons tomato paste

1 tablespoon prepared mustard

1 teaspoon chili powder

2 teaspoons Worcestershire sauce

½ teaspoon salt

½ teaspoon sugar

½ teaspoon dried oregano

⅛ teaspoon ground black pepper

6 hamburger buns

Brown the meat in a large, heated, nonstick skillet. Add the onion and green pepper. Cook 10 more minutes. Stir in tomato sauce and the rest of the ingredients (except the buns). Reduce the heat to medium low, cover, and cook 15 minutes stirring occasionally. Spoon ½ cup of the mixture over the bottom half of each bun; cover with the top half of bun.

Yield: 6 sandwiches

Baked Ziti with Spinach, Tomatoes, and Smoked Mozzarella

This is a great one-dish meal that gives you protein, veggies, and dairy—in just one recipe! Another advantage: you can make this ahead for later, or freeze it for another day.

8 ounces ziti, cooked

1 tablespoon olive oil

1 cup chopped onion

1 cup chopped yellow bell pepper

2 garlic cloves, minced

One 14 ½ -ounce can diced tomatoes with basil, garlic, and oregano

One 10-ounce can Italian seasoned and diced tomatoes (optional)

4 cups baby spinach

1¼ cups (5 ounces) shredded, plain or smoked mozzarella, divided

Cooking spray

Cook pasta according to the package directions, subtracting 2 minutes of cooking time because the pasta will continue to cook in the oven. Do not add salt or fat to the water. Drain and hold until needed.

Preheat oven to 375 degrees.

In a Dutch oven, heat the oil over medium high heat. Add the onion and pepper; sauté for 5 minutes. Add garlic to the pan; sauté for 2 minutes or until the onion is tender. Stir in tomatoes; bring to a boil. Reduce heat; simmer for 5 minutes stirring occasionally. Add spinach to pan; cook 30 seconds or until spinach wilts, stirring frequently. Remove from the heat. Add pasta and ¾ cup of cheese to the tomato mixture. Toss well to combine. Spoon the pasta mixture into an 11 × 7-inch baking dish lightly coated with cooking spray; sprinkle evenly with remaining cheese. Bake at 375 degrees for 15 minutes, or until the cheese melts and begins to brown.

Yield: 6 servings

chapter 10

Ask Dr. Rob:

COMMON QUESTIONS ABOUT FITNESS IN KIDS

Every Saturday morning, I host a sports and fitness show on 1050 ESPN Radio in New York. These are some of the questions I am often asked regarding exercise and sports:

Q: My 8-year-old loves basketball. What can I do to help improve her skills?

A: Always work with her team or friends, and try to make learning fun. Unfortunately, the key to success is found in one boring word: repetition. Kids quickly lose interest unless there's some kind of game attached to a drill, so the secret to improving skill at this stage is to present repetition disguised as a creative, game-like activity. This technique works with boys, too, because at this age there is no great disparity between the endurance and strength of girls and boys.

To practice dribbling, gather a group of kids and demonstrate the rudiments of dribbling in 2 minutes or less. As you know, brevity works because the younger the kid, the shorter the attention span. Once you've explained the fundamentals, arrange two sets of parallel cones and divide the kids into teams. The object of this exercise is to get each team through the cones successfully. The first team to do this twice wins. All you'll have to do is stand back and watch them cheer their teammates to victory. It's good training, and great for team spirit, too.

You can offer a similar challenge with shooting drills. Create two lines of kids, and have each of them stand 5 feet from the basket. Then let them have a shooting contest. The first team to score ten baskets wins.

Always remember that, at this age, only the basic skills should be emphasized: dribbling, passing, shooting, and basic defensive positioning.

Q: My 9-year-old son is limping, and I know he didn't hurt himself. What does this mean?

A: The sudden onset of a limp that is not associated with an injury should send you—immediately—to your pediatrician because it can have many causes. Often the limp indicates a hip problem, the most common of which is *transient synovitis,* a temporary condition that can be the result of a virus or allergy. The outward symptoms can be difficulty in walking and swelling in the hip area. Improvement is rapid with rest and/or age-appropriate anti-inflammatory medication.

Another cause for limping can be *Legg-Calve-Perthes disease,* which is caused by altered blood flow to the hip.

Your pediatrician *must* be consulted, because these possibilities, as well as others such as infection, Lyme disease, or juvenile arthritis, need to be ruled out.

Q: My 11-year-old told me last night that his back hurts. How long should I wait before I see a doctor?

A: Any child who develops back pain that is not the result of an obvious injury requires an immediate medical evaluation.

As a parent, your first job is to help your child recall his recent activities and determine if an injury might be involved. If so, medical evaluation might still be important. The more you can contribute to the doctor's knowledge about possible sources of the pain, the easier it will be for her to help your child. If there are no physical changes after a minor injury, the back pain should disappear within 2 weeks with appropriate rest, ice or heat, and (in some cases) a dose or two of anti-inflammatory medication. Should pain persist beyond 2 weeks, check again with your doctor.

As many as 5 percent of young children have premature wearing of the discs in the spine, causing low back pain, which is why immediate evaluation of back pain not related to a specific injury is required. The prudent physician will also consider other spine-related conditions such as *spondylolisthesis,* a slippage or abnormal movement of one vertebra on another, or *tumors,* which can be accompanied by other signs such as weakness and weight loss.

Q: I don't think the coach of my son's soccer team insists on enough water breaks. What's the rule on this?

A: You're right in wanting the coach to offer water breaks, because kids, unlike adults, don't always recognize thirst. Even if they do, they usually hate calling attention to themselves for something so "baby-like" as a water break. Kids do get dehydrated quickly, however, because they have a relatively small skin area and are more quickly subject to the effects of heat. To avoid dehydration, I recommend that any activity requiring fairly continuous motion, such as soccer, basketball, hockey, and lacrosse, requires a drink break every 15 minutes.

Water is all that is needed for short-duration activities, but a sports drink (one with both carbohydrates and minerals such as sodium and potassium) is preferred if the event lasts more than 1 hour, because these drinks replace both the fluid and electrolytes that are lost in sweating and continuous activity. One-half glass of fluid is recommended for every 15 minutes of continuous physical activity and/or if the temperature is warm. This is especially true for what I call the "80/80 Club," which is when the ambient temperature is above 80 degrees F, and the relative humidity is above 80 percent. Participating in continuous outdoor endurance-type (running) activities is *not* recommended under these conditions.

Q: Our neighbors bought a trampoline, and every time I look out the kitchen window I see five or six kids jumping at the same time. Is this safe?

A: Leave the dishes in the sink, Mom, and run right out there and get those kids off that trampoline. *Basic rule: one kid jumping at a time.* According to the American Association of Orthopedic Surgeons, approximately 250,000 trampoline injuries occur every year in the United States, and those are just the injuries that required medical care. Further, the injured kids are generally under the age of 14, and most are hurt because of improper use of the trampoline. Here are some basic safety rules:

- Trampolines should be located in well-lit areas.
- No one should jump onto the trampoline from a ledge or platform.
- The trampoline jumping surface should be at ground level.
- Supporting bars, strings, and surrounding landing surfaces should be well padded.
- Somersaults and other risky maneuvers should be performed only with proper adult supervision.
- An observing adult should always be present. I am passionate about parental

supervision on the trampoline, pool, beach, and all other places—even when there is a lifeguard present. No one can ever take the place of an eagle-eyed parent.

Q: When my son was born, I was thrilled to think that I'd have someone to shoot baskets with, take to ball games, and take on fishing trips. Now my son is 7, and he hates sports. What can I do to make him like them?

A: Not a blessed thing. You know my philosophy is "Let Kids Be Kids." This means don't be a pushy parent. Sports are not a rite of passage, Dad. Your son can grow up to be an intelligent, mature, caring person even if he never picks up a bat or kicks a soccer ball. Let him do what pleases him—read, play an instrument, or be an actor. Your job as a loving parent is to provide opportunities, wherever possible, for your child to pursue his interests and to encourage him to be the best he can, so his self-esteem remains intact even though he's not the star of the basketball team. It's important, however, to find some form of physical activity to occupy some of his time—perhaps the two of you can play catch using a ball or Frisbee.

Q: One of the girls on our lacrosse team had a slight concussion the other day. The coach suggested that her mother should wake her during the night to be sure that she was okay. Was that the right advice?

A: Sorry to disagree with the coach, but that was not the correct advice. There is no valid reason to awaken a child who has sustained a garden-variety concussion. Contrary to popular belief, a sleeping child who has suffered a concussion is not at increased risk if allowed to remain comfortably at rest. Parents need to keep the child away from contact activities until any symptoms have disappeared. (For more discussion about concussions, see Chapter 6.)

Q: My niece is studying ballet and had to quit this week because she was diagnosed with Osgood-Schlatter syndrome. What's that?

A: It sounds like the name of a German moviemaker, but in reality it is a rather benign, short-term disease. The first symptom is usually pain in the front of the knee just below the kneecap, which might be accompanied by swelling, tenderness, and aching pain. The pain worsens when a child's activity increases, and gets better with rest. This is a common, temporary condition that comes from overuse of the legs. It usually occurs in very active kids between the ages of 8 and 16. It's a common problem for all active sports and—as you now know—for dancers, too.

This condition usually affects only one knee; the symptoms are a slightly swollen, warm and tender bony bump just below the child's kneecap. If you press the bump, your child will say "Owwww."

All that is required is rest for the knee until it gets better, which can be from 6 to 18 months. Before giving your child any medication, check with your physician to make sure it's okay. Your doctor might suggest a pain reliever such as ibuprofen or acetaminophen. When the pain subsides, a good strengthening program might help. Tell your niece's parents to consider icing the area after use of the knee, and ask the doctor to prescribe some stretches to help avoid this problem in the future.

Q: When kids are active in sports, they want snacks, and they don't like big meals that much. What kinds of snacks do you give the kids on your teams?

A: The usual stuff (apples, carrot sticks), but to keep it all interesting, we divide snacks into four categories. Here are some of the things we feed them:

- *Crunchies* such as pretzels, popcorn, trail mix, granola bars, and baked chips
- *Chewies* such as bagels and dried fruit (including raisins)
- *Yummies* such as pudding packs, milk, yogurt, or peanut butter
- *Juicies*, including juice packs, Jell-O packs, canned fruits, and fresh fruit (grapes, oranges)

Q: My 11-year-old daughter plays soccer, and her coach has told the girls that they should be sure to stretch before games to avoid ACL injuries. What does ACL mean?

A: It sounds as if your daughter has a smart coach who knows that girls are more likely to sustain this type of injury, which is a sprain (or rupture) of the anterior cruciate ligament (ACL). The ACL is one of the four main ligaments that connect the thigh bone to the shin bone. Girls and women (rather than boys) usually suffer this injury because of anatomic, biomechanical, and possibly hormonal differences. Experts believe that girls should perform leg muscle strengthening and balance exercises, as well as speed training; make certain they have good footwear and orthotics, if needed; and get instruction on good jumping and landing practices (no straight knee landings, kids).

Q: Do all kids from the ages of 5–12 need vitamin supplements?

A: No, Mom, not every child needs vitamin supplements. Kids who don't eat enough healthy foods do, and so do children diagnosed with specific vitamin deficiencies. But don't stuff your kid with vitamins and think you've done your job. Vitamins, like everything else, are to be used only when and if needed. I urge you to check your local water supply, because the water in many areas does not contain sufficient fluoride, and you will need to supplement in order to meet your growing child's needs.

Q: I took my son to his older brother's tennis match (which he won), and my younger son turned to me and said, "I am never playing tennis, Dad." He is a well-coordinated kid, but I don't think he wants to be compared to his big brother. Any suggestions for athletic involvement for the little guy?

A: Sounds as if he knows what he can handle. I recommend a sport where your son can blend in with a group and doesn't feel pressured to focus on individual performance. Soccer and lacrosse would be optimal for him, because baseball and basketball tend to focus more on the individual performance of batters and shooters. Who knows? Once he starts playing team sports, he might gain the confidence he needs to move on to other activities.

Another good choice is weightlifting, as long as you keep it noncompetitive. Weight training challenges the child and gives him the possibility of improving his own performance. Machine weights are fine; they can be safe, and they isolate specific muscle groups. However, I recommend using free weights, even when machines are available, because they mimic "real life" challenges and work out several related muscle groups. (For more information about weight training, see Chapter 3.)

Q: How much should my daughter drink during her lacrosse game? She says she doesn't like to have water just before she plays.

A: Your daughter, like most kids, isn't truly aware of her need for hydration. I recommend 2–3 glasses of fluid 2–3 hours prior to game time, because fluid takes time to move from the stomach to the intestines, where it is absorbed. She might think this is uncomfortable, so start getting her accustomed to drinking more water during practice. Further, she should have glass of fluid every 15 minutes during play.

To eliminate the possibility that your daughter is afraid she'll have to go to the bathroom in the middle of a game, remind her to go before the game starts and during any breaks in play.

After the game, she should drink 2–3 glasses of a sports drink for both the carbohydrates and minerals. If this seems excessive, remember that there are many positive reasons to be well hydrated. Dehydration can cause fatigue, performance impairment, and heat exhaustion, as well as such serious problems as heat stroke and heart failure. Of course, be careful not to drink too much fluid (over-hydrate). This condition is called *hyponatremia*, and it occurs when a person consumes too much water, thereby diluting the electrolytes in the body. This is why it is important to drink sports drinks in addition to water as part of the rehydration process. Sports drinks replenish electrolytes while also hydrating.

Q: My son's coach doesn't want the kids to have sports drinks. I say they're okay but not mandatory. What do you think?

A: If the game or practice takes less than 60 minutes, plain water is usually just fine. However, if the event is more than 1 hour in length, an 8-ounce sports drink with 6–8 percent carbohydrates and 50–80 calories (almost any commercial one) is appropriate.

A sports drink that contains more than 8 percent sugar (or carbohydrates) will slow absorption and can cause nausea, cramps, and diarrhea. This includes fruit juices and soft drinks.

A few reminders: your child doesn't lose vitamins when he perspires, so don't spend money on sports drinks with added vitamins. Also, cold drinks are not absorbed more quickly than hot drinks, so give kids hot or cold.

Q: Last night, my 9-year-old daughter woke up crying because her legs hurt. Her dad and I rubbed her legs. He wanted to give her acetaminophen, but I didn't know whether it was appropriate. What do you think?

A: Your daughter was probably experiencing "growing pains." About 25 percent of all kids experience similar symptoms of this benign condition. It usually occurs in early childhood (ages 3–5) and again a few years later (ages 8–11), because these are the times of active growth spurts. One way to diagnose growing pains is if the area feels better when rubbed or massaged. If there is a more serious problem, rubbing might increase the discomfort. See your doctor if the pain is accompanied by fever, a rash, loss of appetite, weakness, fatigue, or a limp.

The best treatment for growing pains is just to be a supportive parent. Acetaminophen (Tylenol®) or ibuprofen (Advil®) can be given to alleviate her discomfort. Massage, stretching, and warming the area can also help reduce the pain. There is no proof that bone growth causes pain, and the discomfort is usually experienced by more active kids as a result of running, jumping, and other activities. Growing pains are felt in the muscles, not the joints. Still, if you are in doubt about the source of the pain, consult a physician so that any worrisome health problems can be eliminated

Q: My kids aren't rough players, but—like all kids—they sometimes come home with abrasions on their knees, elbows, or thighs. What should I do?
A: Clean the area with lots of water and cleansing soap. Then apply a thin layer of an antibacterial ointment. Before applying the ointment (or any medication), I recommend that you always check the ingredients on the label to make sure there are no possible allergic reactions for the child. Also, make sure the product has not passed its expiration date. It's also a good idea to keep wounds lightly covered with a clean, sterile gauze. Tell the child to keep the area clean and out of play for a few days. If the area begins to exude pus or a fever develops, seek medical care.

Q: My son plays on a Little League team, and he is probably the best base runner on the team. His coach wants him to slide head first. I think this is asking for trouble. Shouldn't a 10-year-old slide feet first?
A: Most coaches and athletes agree that head first is best, but researchers claim there is no real difference in time in getting to the base. When it comes to safety, more injuries probably occur sliding in feet first. However, foot and ankle injuries, which are typical feet-first injuries, are generally less serious than the head or neck injuries that can occur with head-first slides. So, the answer to your question is: it depends.

The most important factor is proper technique coupled with good body mechanics. Some players wear wrist guards in addition to ankle, shin, and elbow guards, as well as batting helmets. Check and see if your team is using breakaway bases, which are held in place by magnets or Velcro™ and decrease the possibility of injuries when the player slides feet first. Another caution: tell your sliding son to always wear long pants. Kids who play in shorts get more frequent cuts and scrapes. The final answer: slide, kid, slide—and do it the way you've practiced, practiced, practiced.

Q: My son hates sports, but I feel that I should push him to play because he needs the exercise. Is this true?

A: Absolutely *not*. Pushing your child into an activity he hates will likely not only be unsuccessful; it might totally turn him off to exercise and create friction between you and him. There seems to be a myth that it is a rite of passage for all kids to play sports, which is not true—although all kids do need to exercise. Any activity that gives a child 30–40 minutes of aerobic activity at least 3–4 days a week is good. This could be a game of tag with friends, a brisk walk with the family dog, or a bike ride. There are many other recreational activities for kids to enjoy, including martial arts, music lessons, and gymnastics classes.

Q: My daughter is worried about eating before her school basketball game. How much rest does she need between eating and game time?

A: There are many opinions about this. Many people believe that it takes about 60 minutes to clear food from the stomach before team play. However, if your daughter is going to participate in an endurance event such as a marathon race, she should allow 2 hours.

Q: Are there days when it's just too hot to play sports?

A: When the ambient temperature and relative humidity are both above 80, hold the outdoor activities. Urge the kids to find a cool, shaded area, and give them plenty of fluids (at least ½ glass for every 15 minutes of activity in extremes of temperature and humidity). A sports drink or water is adequate if the activity lasts less than 45 minutes. For activities lasting longer than this, a sport drink is recommended.

Q: The school nurse told Timmy he just has "a little ankle sprain," and that he could play sports on the sprained ankle. Do you agree?

A: Strangely enough, it's okay to move about freely with minor sprains and strains—

if the child can bear weight on the limb with minimal to no pain. However, a sprain might be significant if the ankle is swollen and bearing weight is difficult. A serious sprain can take 3–6 weeks to heal. If you're in doubt about the seriousness of the sprain, do what all concerned parents do, and take Timmy to the doctor.

Q: My 10-year-old son has begun to weight train and wants to start drinking protein shakes. Is this okay?

A: Protein powder drinks have become an epidemic fad throughout the country. They are touted as essential requirements to repair damaged muscles in people who weight train. Actually, most children consume more than enough protein in a regular, healthy diet to sustain adequate growth *and* repair injured muscles. The reference chart on page 72 lists the guidelines for protein requirements throughout growth and development. Simply keep a record of the child's diet for a week or so, and you will see if your child is consuming adequate protein (see Appendix B).

Q: My child has just entered middle school, and one of the older kids suggested he start taking creatine to build muscle strength. Can this supplement damage his kidneys?

A: I wish I could unequivocally say "Yes." But even though I can't, I strongly urge you to prevent your child from using creatine. This supplement works by increasing the water content of muscles, thereby enlarging them. However, medical science is still debating the side effects of creatine. Its effect on the heart, which is also a muscle, is still unknown. It does cause bloating, and there is a possible link with kidney stone formation. There's no better way to gain muscle mass than the good old-fashioned way: hard work.

Q: Whenever my child plays soccer, she seems to get light-headed and exhausted even though she drinks plenty of water. What could be wrong?

A: Of course, the first thing you need to do is take her to the pediatrician for an evaluation. Several conditions may be present. Certainly, plain old fatigue is a possible cause. She might also be hypoglycemic. After a certain amount of activity, the blood sugar can drop, causing the symptoms you mention. The pediatrician will order blood tests and likely a glucose-tolerance test. If no clear-cut sugar condition is identified, following the glycemic index (GI) of certain foods might help resolve some of these symptoms. This index is a guide to the available sugar content of food. Foods with a higher GI make sugar readily available as soon as they are consumed. These foods are good for short bursts of energy. Foods with a low GI release sugars more slowly into the bloodstream; these foods are better for endurance activities, including marathon races or long competitions such as a soccer game (see Resources section).

Hopefully, your questions have been answered. However, as a doctor who is faced with new challenges every day, I am sure you'll think of at least one question I've never heard before.

Fortunately, I'm just an e-mail away. Address your questions to me at my website, www.drrobsays.com, and before you know it, you'll have the answer you need. Meanwhile—live healthy.

chapter 11

where do we go from here, dr. rob?

Okay, I've learned a lot about getting my child up and moving and eat right. Where do we go from here? Your next step depends on your child. If you're hoping you can send your kid to college on a sports scholarship, my best advice is to talk to the school advisors. If you're asking "where do we go from here" because you are amazed by the amount of money ballplayers get just for signing a contract, you might have overly high expectations for your child. A word of caution: only 1 percent of children go on to have successful professional sporting careers, but nearly 100 percent can achieve better health through sports and exercise.

Some kids play football; some kids *are* the football. The child's emotions and accomplishments are kicked, tossed, and discussed, as he becomes the center of family life. As a result, kids often attempt to win their parents' approval by scoring one more goal, getting one more "A," or adding one more extracurricular activity.

⇨ *It's time that all parents stopped living or reliving their lives through their children. Children do not need wall-to-wall activities; they need time to play. YES, PLAY!*

Your friends might brag about "my kid, the third baseman," or "my daughter, who takes dance and music and drama; she has the lead in the school play; and she is a cheerleader and gets good grades." My favorite is, "Dr. Rob, my son hurt his arm when he won his tennis tournament, and the pain is pretty intense." In all my years of medical interviewing, I do not recall ever asking whether a child won or lost while sustaining an injury, yet so many parents are eager to tell me about their star athletes. How many parents talk about "my kid, who has ulcers"? When was the last time someone said, "Did I tell you about my daughter's depression? Bulimia? Weight problem?"

For those of you who swear your budding superstar is the real deal, let me deflate your bubble: even if he is, it's very unlikely that what you see now will blossom into something really serious in 5 years. In fact, my biggest concern is not false ideations, but rather the young budding superstars who actually believe the praise they get from mom and dad. I'm concerned for the kid who actually buys into the idea that he is the "best of the best." Then, one day, poof, a deflated ego and depressed personality invade his mindset. Realization sets in. Little Timmy isn't that superstar mom and dad kept talking about; in fact, he's just another kid.

Your home is the breeding ground for your child's future. The sense of security given to the boy who knows his parents love him unconditionally, or the girl who doesn't have to perform on stage to win a parent's applause, is the greatest gift a parent can give to a child.

We need to accept our children for what they are *not*, as well as for what they *are*. Encouraging a child doesn't mean pushing her from the crib to stardom in the one area where *you* always wanted to excel.

As parents, we need to relax with our kids and let them move at their own pace and at their own level. We need to listen to them and help where and when we can.

Yet, we can never be too careful in supervising their safe play. Who ever said parenting was going to be easy?

Sports can lead to physical, psychological, and social health and well-being. Along the way, sports also can help with special problems.

Overweight child? That child needs both the exercise and commitment that sports requires. Child with a short attention span? Sports can enhance focus and concentration.

It doesn't have to be organized sports. It can be playing outside with the kids in the neighborhood, roller-blading, or bike riding—whatever makes a child feel a sense of accomplishment and satisfaction.

Sports can be fun, and since childhood is a short time in a long life, let's just relax and let kids be kids.

⇨ *Remember:*

Success breeds confidence and confidence breeds success!

General

Food pyramid: www.mypyramid.gov.
Glycemic index: www.mendosa.com
Protein available from various food sources: http://www.nwhealth.edu/healthyU/
eatWell/protein3.html

Medical Societies and Organizations

American Medical Association
www.ama-assn.org

American Academy of Pediatrics
www.aap.org

American Pediatric Society and Society of Pediatric Research
www.aps-spr.org

American College of Sports Medicine
www.acsm.org

American Heart Association
www.americanheart.org

American Diabetes Association
www.diabetes.org

American Dietetic Association
www.eatright.org

American Academy of Asthma, Allergy and Immunology
www.aaaai.org

Youth Sports and Fitness Organizations

National Alliance for Youth Sports
www.nays.org
(800) 688-KIDS

National Youth Sports Safety Foundation
www.nyssf.org

American Fitness Alliance (Youth Fitness Resource Center)
www.americanfitness.net

Youth Information for Moms
www.momsteam.com

National Youth Sports Coaches Association
www.nays.org

General Safety

I'm Safe Network
(provides information to children so that they make s
mart choices and avoid unintentional injury)
www.imsafe.com

Consumer.gov
Access federal consumer information, including the
Consumer Action Handbook, scam alerts, and recent bulletins.
www.consumer.gov

Consumer Product Safety Commission
Federal agency works to help keep families safe by
reducing risks of injury or death from consumer products.
www.cpsc.gov

Consumer Product Safety Commission - Kidd Safety
Check out interactive games for kids dealing with safety.
Includes safety tips for fireworks and bike riding.
www.cpsc.gov/kids/kidsafety

U.S. Consumer Product Safety Commission – Kid Safety
Aims to educate the public about safety issues related to
consumer products for kids. Includes bikes, scooters, and toys.
www.cpsc.gov/kids/kidsafety/index.html

More Websites

www.bam.gov

www.kidshealth.org

www.momsteam.org

www.thecenterforkidsfirst.org

www.presidentschallenge.org

www.diabetesnet.com

www.dietitian.com

KidsMeds:
providing pediatric drug information to parents
www.kidsmeds.com

Rehabilitation and Children with Special Needs
(for child health information and agencies addressing disability issues)
www.ems-c.org/rehab/framerehab.htm

weight/volume equivalents for the major food groups

FROM HTTP://WWW.MYPYRAMID.GOV/PYRAMID/INDEX.HTML

WHAT COUNTS AS 1 CUP IN THE MILK GROUP?

The chart lists specific amounts that count as 1 cup in the milk group toward your daily recommended intake:

	Amount that counts as 1 cup in the milk group	Common portions and cup equivalents
Milk *[choose fat-free or low-fat milk most often]*	1 cup 1 half-pint container ½ cup evaporated milk	
Yogurt *[choose fat-free or low-fat yogurt most often]*	1 regular container (8 fluid ounces)	1 small container (6 ounces) = ¾ cup
	1 cup	1 snack size container (4 ounces) = ½ cup

Cheese *[choose low-fat* *cheeses most often]*	1½ ounces hard cheese (cheddar, mozzarella, Swiss, parmesan)	1 slice of hard cheese is equivalent to ½ cup milk
	⅓ cup shredded cheese	
	2 ounces processed cheese (American)	1 slice of processed cheese is equivalent to ⅓ cup milk
	½ cup ricotta cheese	
	2 cups cottage cheese	½ cup cottage cheese is equivalent to ¼ cup milk
Milk-based desserts *[choose fat-free or* *low-fat types most often]*	1 cup pudding made with milk 1 cup frozen yogurt	
	1½ cups ice cream	1 scoop ice cream is equivalent to ⅓ cup milk

WHAT COUNTS AS A 1-OUNCE EQUIVALENT IN THE MEAT & BEANS GROUP?

In general, 1 ounce of meat, poultry, or fish; ¼ cup cooked dry beans; 1 egg; 1 tablespoon of peanut butter; or ½ ounce of nuts or seeds can be considered as a 1-ounce equivalent from the meat and beans group.

The chart lists specific amounts that count as a 1-ounce equivalent in the Meat and Beans group toward your daily recommended intake:

	Amount that counts as 1 ounce equivalent in the Meat and Beans group	Common portions and ounce equivalents
Meats	1 ounce cooked lean beef	1 small steak (eye of round, filet) = 3½ to 4 ounce equivalents
	1 ounce cooked lean pork or ham	1 small lean hamburger = 2 to 3 ounce equivalents
Poultry	1 ounce cooked chicken or turkey, without skin	1 small chicken breast half = 3 ounce equivalents
	1 sandwich slice of turkey (4½ x 2½ x ⅛-inch)	½ Cornish game hen = 4 ounce equivalents
Fish	1 ounce cooked fish or shell fish	1 can of tuna, drained = 3 to 4ounce equivalents 1 salmon steak = 4 to 6 ounce equivalents 1 small trout = 3 ounce equivalents
Eggs	1 egg	
Nuts and seeds	½ ounce of nuts (12 almonds, 24 pistachios, 7 walnut halves)	1 ounce of nuts or seeds = 2 oz equivalents

½ ounce of seeds (pumpkin,
sunflower or squash seeds,
hulled, roasted)

1 tablespoon of peanut butter
or almond butter

Dry beans and peas	¼ cup of cooked dry beans (such as black, kidney, pinto, or white beans)	1 cup split pea soup = 2 oz eq 1 cup lentil soup = 2 oz eq 1 cup bean soup = 2 oz eq
	¼ cup of cooked dry peas (such as chickpeas, cowpeas, lentils, or split peas)	
	¼ cup of baked beans, refried beans	
	¼ cup (about 2 ounces) of tofu patty = 2 oz eq	1 soy or bean burger
	1 ounce tempeh, cooked ¼ cup roasted soybeans 1 falafel patty (2¼-inch, 4-ounce) 2 tablespoon hummus	

WHAT COUNTS AS A CUP OF FRUIT?

In general, 1 cup of fruit, 100-percent fruit juice, or ½ cup of dried fruit can be considered as 1 cup from the fruit group. The following specific amounts count as 1 cup of fruit (in some cases, equivalents for ½ cup are also shown) toward your daily recommended intake:

	Amount that counts as 1 cup of fruit	Amount that counts as ½ cup of fruit
Apple or	½ large (3.25" diameter) 1 cup sliced or chopped, raw or cooked	1 small (2.5" diameter) ½ cup sliced or chopped, raw cooked
Applesauce	1 cup	1 snack container (4 ounce)
Banana long)	1 cup sliced 1 large (8 to 9 inches long)	1 small (less than 6 inches
Cantaloupe med.	1 cup diced or melon balls melon)	1 medium wedge (⅛ of a
Grapes	1 cup whole or cut-up 32 seedless grapes	16 seedless grapes
Grapefruit	1 medium (4-inch diameter) 1 cup sections	½ medium (4-inch diameter)
Mixed fruit (fruit cocktail)	1 cup diced or sliced, raw, or canned, drained	1 snack container (4-ounce) drained = ⅜ cup
Orange	1 large (3 1/16-inch diameter) 1 cup sections	1 small (2⅜-inch diameter)
Orange, mandarin	1 cup canned, drained	

Peach	1 large (2¾-inch diameter) 1 cup sliced or diced, raw, cooked, or canned, drained 2 halves, canned	1 small (2-inch diameter) 1 snack container (4-ounce) drained = ⅜ cup
Pear	1 medium pear (2.5 per pound) 1 cup sliced or diced, raw, cooked, or canned, drained	1 snack container (4-ounce) drained = ⅜ cup
Pineapple	1 cup chunks, sliced or crushed, raw, cooked or canned, drained	1 snack container (4-ounce) drained = ⅜ cup
Plum	1 cup sliced raw or cooked 3 medium or 2 large plums	1 large plum
Strawberries sliced	About 8 large berries 1 cup whole, halved, or sliced,	½ cup whole, halved, or fresh or frozen
Watermelon	1 small wedge (1-inch thick) 1 cup diced or balls	6 melon balls
Dried fruit (raisins, prunes, apricots, etc.)	½ cup dried fruit is equivalent to 1 cup fruit, ½ cup raisins, ½ cup prunes ½ cup dried apricots	¼ cup dried fruit is equivalent to ½ cup fruit; 1 small box raisins (1.5-ounce)
100-percent fruit juice (orange, apple, grape, grapefruit, etc.)	1 cup	½ cup

WHAT COUNTS AS A CUP OF VEGETABLES?

In general, 1 cup of raw or cooked vegetables or vegetable juice, or 2 cups of raw leafy greens can be considered as 1 cup from the vegetable group. The chart lists specific amounts that count as 1 cup of vegetables (in some cases equivalents for ½ cup are also shown) toward your recommended intake:

	AMOUNT THAT COUNTS AS 1 CUP OF VEGETABLES	AMOUNT THAT COUNTS AS ½ CUP OF VEGETABLES
Dark-Green Vegetables		
Broccoli	1 cup chopped or florets 3 spears 5-inch long raw or cooked	
Greens, (collards mustard greens, turnip greens, kale)	1 cup cooked	
Spinach	1 cup, cooked 2 cups raw is equivalent to 1 cup of vegetables	1 cup raw is equivalent to ½ cup of vegetables
Raw leafy greens: Spinach, romaine, watercress, dark green leafy lettuce, endive, escarole	2 cups raw is equivalent to 1 cup of vegetables	1 cup raw is equivalent to 1½ cup of vegetables
Orange Vegetables		
Carrots	1 cup, strips, slices, or chopped, raw or cooked	
	2 medium	1 medium carrot
	1 cup baby carrots (about 12)	About 6 baby carrots

Pumpkin	1 cup mashed, cooked	
Sweet potato	1 large baked (2¼-inch or more diameter) 1 cup sliced, or mashed, cooked	
Winter squash (acorn, butternut, hubbard)	1 cup cubed, cooked	½ acorn squash, baked = ¾ cup

Dry beans and peas

Dry beans and peas (such as black, garbanzo, kidney, pinto, or soy beans, or black eyed peas or split peas)	1 cup whole or mashed, cooked	
Tofu	1 cup ½-inch cubes (about 8 ounces)	1 piece 2½ x 2¾ x 1-inch (about 4 ounces)

Starchy Vegetables

Corn, yellow or white	1 cup	
	1 large ear (8 to 9 inches long)	1 small ear (about 6 inches long)
Green peas	1 cup	
White potatoes	1 cup diced, mashed	
	1 medium boiled or baked potato (2½ to 3-inch diameter)	
	French fried: 20 medium to long strips (2½ to 4 inches long) (Contains discretionary calories.)	

	AMOUNT THAT COUNTS AS 1 CUP OF VEGETABLES	AMOUNT THAT COUNTS AS ½ CUP OF VEGETABLES
Other Vegetables		
Bean sprouts	1 cup cooked	
Cabbage, green	1 cup, chopped or shredded, raw or cooked	
Cauliflower	1 cup pieces or florets raw or cooked	
Celery	1 cup, diced or sliced, raw or cooked	
	2 large stalks (11 to 12 inches long)	1 large stalk (11 to 12 inches long)
Cucumbers or chopped	1 cup raw, sliced	
Green or wax beans	1 cup cooked	
Green or red peppers	1 cup chopped, raw or cooked	
	1 large pepper (3-inch diameter, 3¾ inches long)	1 small pepper
Lettuce, iceberg or head	2 cups raw, shredded or chopped = equivalent to 1 cup of vegetables	1 cup raw, shredded or chopped = equivalent to ½ cup of vegetables
Mushrooms	1 cup raw or cooked	
Onions	1 cup chopped, raw or cooked	
Tomatoes	1 large raw whole (3-inch)	1 small raw whole (2¼-inch)
	1 cup chopped or sliced, raw, canned, or cooked	1 medium canned

Tomato or mixed vegetable juice	1 cup		½ cup
Summer squash or zucchini	1 cup cooked, sliced or diced		

WHAT COUNTS AS AN OUNCE EQUIVALENT OF GRAINS?

In general, 1 slice of bread, 1 cup of ready-to-eat cereal, or ½ cup of cooked rice, cooked pasta, or cooked cereal can be considered as a 1-ounce equivalent from the grains group.

The chart lists specific amounts that count as 1-ounce equivalent of grains toward your daily recommended intake. In some cases, the number of ounce equivalents for common portions are also shown.

		Amount that counts as 1 ounce equivalent of grains	Common portions and ounce equivalents
Bagels	WG*: Whole-wheat RG*: Plain, egg	1 "mini" bagel = 4 ounce equivalents	1 large bagel
Biscuits	(Baking powder/ buttermilk—RG*)	1 small (2-inch diameter)	1 large (3-inch diameter) = 2 ounce equivalents
Breads	WG*: 100% Whole-wheat RG*: White, wheat, French, sourdough	1 regular slice 1 small slice French 4 snack-size slices rye bread	2 regular slices = 2 ounce equivalents
Bulgur	Cracked wheat (WG*)	½ cup cooked	
Cornbread	(RG*)	1 small piece (2 ½ x 1¼ x 1¼-inch)	1 medium piece (2½ x 2½ x 1¼-inch) = 2 ounce equivalents

Crackers	WG*: 100% whole-wheat, rye	5 whole-wheat crackers 2 rye crisp breads	
	RG*: Saltines, snack crackers	7 square or round crackers	
English muffins	WG*: Whole-wheat RG*: Plain, raisin	½ muffin	1 muffin = 2 ounce equivalents
Muffins	WG*: Whole-wheat RG*: Bran, corn, plain)	1 small (2½-inch diameter	1 large (3½-inch diameter) = 3 ounce equivalents
Oatmeal	(WG)	½ cup cooked 1 packet instant 1 ounce dry (regular or quick)	
Pancakes	WG*: Whole-wheat, buckwheat RG*: Buttermilk, plain	1 pancake (4½-inch diameter) 2 small pancakes (3-inch diameter)	3 pancakes (4½-inch diameter) = 3 ounce equivalents
Popcorn	(WG*)	3 cups, popped	1 microwave bag, popped = 4 ounce equivalents
Ready-to-eat breakfast cereal	WG*: Toasted oat, whole-wheat flakes RG*: Corn flakes, puffed rice	1 cup flakes or rounds 1¼ cup puffed	
Rice	WG*: Brown, wild RG*: Enriched, white, polished	½ cup cooked 1 ounce dry	1 cup cooked = 2 ounce equivalents

Pasta: Spaghetti, macaroni, noodles	WG*: Whole-wheat RG*: Enriched, durum	½ cup cooked 1 ounce dry	1 cup cooked = 2 ounce equivalents
Tortillas	WG*: Whole-wheat, whole-grain corn RG*: Flour, corn)	1 small flour tortilla (6-inch diameter) 1 corn tortilla (6-inch diameter)	1 large tortilla (12-inch diameter) = 4 ounce equivalents

*WG, whole grains; RG, refined grains. This is shown when products are available both in whole-grain and refined-grain forms.

How do I count the oils I eat?

This chart gives a quick guide to the amount of oils in some common foods:

	Amount of food	Amount of oil Teaspoons /grams	Calories from oil Approximate calories	Total calories Approximate calories
Oils:				
Vegetable oils (such as canola, corn, cottonseed, olive, peanut, safflower, soybean, and sunflower)	1 Tbsp	3 tsp/14 g	120	120
Foods rich in oils:				
Margarine, soft (trans fat free)	1 Tbsp	2 ½ tsp/11 g	100	100
Mayonnaise	1 Tbsp	2 ½ tsp/11 g	100	100

Mayonnaise-type salad dressing	1 Tbsp	1 tsp/5 g	45	55
Italian dressing	2 Tbsp	2 tsp/8 g	75	85
Thousand Island dressing	2 Tbsp	2 ½ tsp/11 g	100	120
Olives, ripe, canned	4 large	½ tsp/ 2 g	15	20
Avocado*	½ med	3 tsp/15 g	130	160
Peanut butter*	2 T	4 tsp/ 16 g	140	190
Peanuts, dry roasted*	1 oz	3 tsp/14 g	120	165
Mixed nuts, dry roasted*	1 oz	3 tsp/15 g	130	170
Cashews, dry roasted*	1 oz	3 tsp/13 g	115	165
Almonds, dry roasted*	1 oz	3 tsp/15 g	130	170
Hazelnuts*	1 oz	4 tsp/18 g	160	185
Sunflower seeds*	1 oz	3 tsp/14 g	120	165

index

Note: Boldface numbers indicate illustrations; a *t* indicates a table; and an *r* indicates a recipe.